HAPPY DOWN BELOW

HAPPY
DOWN
BELOW

Everything You Want to Know about the Penis and Other Bits

DR. OLIVER GRALLA

Translated by Jamie McIntosh

FOREWORD BY PETER MOORE

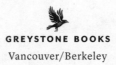

GREYSTONE BOOKS

Vancouver/Berkeley

18 19 20 21 22   5 4 3 2 1

Greystone Books Ltd.
www.greystonebooks.com

Cataloguing data available from Library and Archives Canada
ISBN 978-1-77164-328-3 (pbk.)
ISBN 978-1-77164-329-0 (epub)

Editing by Stephanie Fysh
Cover illustration and design by Brian Tong
Text design by Nayeli Jimenez
Typesetting by Shed Simas / Onça Design
Printed and bound in Canada on ancient-forest-friendly paper by Friesens

We gratefully acknowledge the support of the Canada Council for the Arts, the British Columbia Arts Council, the Province of British Columbia through the Book Publishing Tax Credit, and the Government of Canada for our publishing activities.

Canada

BRITISH COLUMBIA | BRITISH COLUMBIA ARTS COUNCIL
An agency of the Province of British Columbia

Canada Council   Conseil des arts
for the Arts   du Canada

CONTENTS

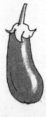

FOREWORD

A T A PIVOTAL point in my journalism career, I quit my job as articles editor for *Playboy*, where I edited serious journalism *and* Playmate data sheets, to become managing editor of *Men's Health*, which included many fewer naked ladies in its editorial pages. My male friends couldn't understand why I'd exchange a clearly ideal job—one that included screening potential Playmates and interviewing the winners—to work for a magazine that often had a half-naked dude on the cover.

But the job switch made sense to *me*, at least. I was just then entering my late thirties, a time of life when all sorts of health concerns crop up.

Why do I suddenly have a potbelly?

Why am I losing my hair?

Am I doomed to the same health maladies as the older men in my family?

And of course, is it safe to stick a pine bough up my urethra?

Actually, that last one wasn't among *my* personal health concerns. But it *was* a question that one of Dr. Gralla's many interesting patients should have taken more seriously before he customized his own Yule log. You'll read all about it in the last chapter. (Spoiler alert: *Don't do it!*)

At *Men's Health*, we took the male organ very seriously indeed, but with the magazine's signature mix of humor and hard science. To educate our millions of penis-owning readers, we even invented our own staff urologist, who, being fictional, possessed none of Dr. Gralla's impressive credentials. But he ably separated phallus fact from dick fiction. We called him Dr. Schwantz, in a nod to our twenty-seven Yiddish-fluent readers (out of five million), who knew the word as slang for a limp male member.

If you're a man, nothing will get your attention like a willie that won't wonka—that won't, with a little encouragement, turn from molten chocolate into a candy bar. This is among the reasons this book belongs in the toolbox of nearly every guy on the planet, plus the women who love them. In fact, many guys don't conduct a downward investigative glance unless our glans is spurting blood, oozing white stuff, pointing listlessly at the floor, or sprouting a tree branch. For all of those conditions and more, Dr. Gralla has nonjudgmental, no-nonsense recommendations, and he deserves our sincere thanks.

But for a moment, let me address all of those problems—except the piney one—from the perspective of a health editor. Over the course of my two-decade stint at *Men's Health*, I came to think of the penis as a very sensitive diagnostic tool. In fact, most men's health scourges—heart disease, diabetes, obesity, psychological problems—manifest themselves early on as dick disorders. Your penis is very likely to know something is wrong before you, your doctor, or even your shrink identifies the malady.

So listen to Dr. Johnson!

If your dick is pointing up, your health is probably pretty good. If it's relentlessly pointing down, so, likely, are your health prospects. All guys have been gifted with an analog wellness meter tucked away in our shorts, to tell us everything we need to know about our schlong-term health prognoses.

Pay attention to the direction yours is pointing, or pay the price. Or, better still, pay a visit to Dr. Gralla's engaging, entertaining text, and get your man-needle pointing northward, pronto.

And while I have your attention, and a sexual soapbox for a moment, I want to call attention to one pet peeve about the male unit that is ably represented by what Dr. Gralla *couldn't* include in this book. There are many helpful pages here devoted to ways to address erectile dysfunction and premature ejaculation—the stalking horses for urology practices everywhere—but few devoted to male birth control options, one of which is to dip your scrotum into scalding water. When the most recent revolutionizer of male birth-control options was Charles Goodyear—the tire guy who invented vulcanized rubber in the 1840s—we are well overdue for the *next* sexual revolution.

Women who don't wish to become pregnant have hundreds of shots, IUDs, sponges, pills, inserts, and potions available at the drop of a prescription. Guys not wanting to get someone pregnant have abstinence, early withdrawal, condoms, and the knife at their disposal. In fact, men have very few options for changing the plotline of *From Here to Paternity*. A male pill, please, and pronto!

But for everything else, there's *Happy Down Below*. Treat yourself and your man-root to a thorough and often uproarious read-through. Your health prospects will be pointing at the ceiling in no time.

—Peter Moore, editor, *Men's Health*, 1995–2015

PREFACE

CTUALLY, I WANTED to be a surgeon. At the age of fifteen, I stood next to my father in an operating theater and, with a heroic expression on my face and an iron hook in my hand, held open the stomach of the patient my father was operating on. You will have noticed: medicine is in my blood. I completed my medical studies with bubbly enthusiasm. On the basis of my thesis, and after my first tentative steps in Hamburg University's Department of Surgery, I was given a scholarship to Harvard University and spent a year in Boston, the mecca of medical science. After careful consideration, however, I opted for quality of life over heroism, and in short order surgery became urology: the specialty that focuses on the urinary system. It was one of the best decisions in my life. Urology is actually the pinnacle of medical science—it's just that hardly anyone realizes it.

For some years now I've been settled in Cologne, Germany, as a urologist, with my main focus on andrology: men's health. At least half of my new patients begin our session with "I've never been to a urologist." I have no idea whether this is an explanation, an apology, or a confession. At any rate, time after time, it astonishes me how little people know about things "down below." Yet it's hardly surprising that mistaken fears and wrong ideas, misunderstandings, and ignorance circulate among my fellow males of all ages. The top 5 issues in the andrological hit parade are erectile dysfunction, premature ejaculation, testosterone, infertility, and male contraception. Women form a subset of our practice, with, for instance, hard-to-treat bladder infections. Over the years, we've developed specific expertise that can make the lives of both men and women a little bit more bearable.

Happy Down Below has one goal: to share a basic understanding and tools of the trade of the perennial problems of urology, thus offering a helping hand on the path back to enjoyment of life. It does this in a way that's easily digestible for every man (and, of course, woman). Some of the many bizarre, curious, and simply odd stories recalled by me and my colleagues in Hamburg's and Cologne's university clinics and in Berlin's Charité medical center have also found their way into the book, to both educate and entertain. I've included pharmacological, orthomolecular, and psychosomatic treatment strategies for individual sectors. But there are also plenty of practical, everyday tips and tricks to be found in this andrological treasure chest. Maybe it could even spare the occasional patient a trip to the andrologist—although, of course, professional expertise can't hurt...

one

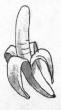

THE UNKNOWN PENIS

EVERY DAY WE hold it in our hand—well, half of us do, at least. Every day. Multiple times a day. As we have for years... decades. A thing of beauty it is *not*, the penis, when it dangles there limp and wrinkled like an old dachshund awkwardly tottering down the stairs, or an organic cucumber, slightly lost behind the carrots at the vegetable stall. Carrots are another thing entirely. And when the penis becomes a firm carrot, it is too. Magnificent erections have always affected the world: inspired art, caused wars, started and ended relationships. Enthusiasm for the magnificence and glory of men's tackle is well within the bounds of my job, not to mention mutual appreciation. So I find it surprising that many men's relationship to their pride and joy alternates between amiable benevolence and complete disinterest. As long as everything works, that's okay, but God help you if there's a problem.

More than once I've wanted to exclaim to a patient encouragingly, "Allow me to introduce you: Your penis"—especially when, once again, someone is standing in front of me dolefully explaining his diagnosis of his narrow foreskin: "I just don't seem to be able to pull it back. It's way too tight. If I try, it's incredibly painful . . . awful. It's been this way for years—well, actually, always. My wife can't stand hearing about it anymore. But can anything be done about it?" Then, as I usually suspect is coming, he adds a proposed treatment: "Can it be operated on?" I purse my lips, tilt my head slightly (usually to the left), and remark in as friendly a way as I can, "Right, then, let's take a look." We go into my examining room next door—couch, ultrasound, swabs. The silicone breast, surely ripe for an Oscar nomination, is stowed away in a drawer, but more on that later.

Now to the "marriage." If this were the auto industry, the process would be described something like the chassis and motor blending to a unity. In my practice man and penis are united. Of course, in the process of demonstrating this, a number of rules must be observed. The most important is that the patient's hands are not allowed to touch his penis. This has proven to be best accomplished by asking the patient to lie on his hands during the examination—my urological handcuffs. The next step: "Close your eyes and think of something pleasant." Usually I ask him to think of a dream destination for his next vacation or the last concert he went to. When the foreskin-afflicted patient is in raptures about Bora Bora, Bruce Springsteen, or Beethoven's Fifth, the magic happens: I pull back the foreskin. And that's it. Not a sound from the patient. No moaning, no hurried prayer, not even an "ouch." I've also got nothing special to report about the penis the foreskin is attached to—not too narrow, no inflammation, not even a trace of redness … just a penis. A bit of soapy water, and all is well. And there it is, the glans, popping out of the foreskin in my thick fingers. There was once a blind Canadian blues singer named Jeff Healey, who died far too young. One of his songs is called "See the Light." The tune always comes to me when, in an examination, a glans first sees the light of day. You may have noticed, urologists have a soft spot for self-pity—especially when it's skillfully presented.

The foreskin slips smoothly again. Everything is hunky-dory, isn't it? What really worries me is a totally different question: Why on earth does someone voluntarily come to me to pull back his foreskin? Just for fun? There are certainly more pleasant things to do in this world. The downcast look, the sweat on the forehead, the fiddling about until the glans is finally freed on the examination couch are evidence of a deeply anchored genuine discomfort. By the way, it was during an examination like this one that the idea of writing this book came to me.

I have the impression that many men invest a lot of money in software but have next to no idea about hardware. Software is the jumble of style, bearing, and status symbols that define our external appearance. Right now it seems that half of men under thirty are wandering around with beards, preferably goatees—the longer, the more masculine. Fancy cars are no longer politically correct or affordable, so instead men are choosing to decorate their faces. I, too, have a beard and drive a Nissan. But for the young beaus of today, what's the chin curtain supposed to be compensating for? As an armchair psychologist, I have a pet theory that many young people from this and the previous generation have had little chance in the early infant stages of their development to become acquainted with their masculine hardware. After Mum's breasts right until preschool it was still predominantly Mum—Dad was at work or not as involved in childcare. In preschools and in elementary schools, they had female teachers. Then suddenly they were twelve and had been through practically all the Freudian development stages without having had a single role model with Y chromosomes. It may well be that this is a bit of a simplification, and I'm not so sure if a Viennese psychiatrist is still the be-all and end-all of cognitive–genital development nowadays. Nevertheless, at the various psychosomatic and sexual therapy symposia and seminars I stumble into from time to time, I hear that during the early development of our sons, male role models are increasingly rare.

But back to Mr. Freud. The phallic phase, the time when we men should become intimately acquainted with our penises, begins around the tender age of five. Don't get me wrong—I'm a big fan of preschools, childcare, and other such setups—but can we not be shown at that age how to pee while standing? The works, including pulling back the foreskin, aiming, and, on completion, packing everything tidily away. It doesn't have to be perfectly done straight off. (And don't forget the handwashing.) Maybe it wouldn't be too bad at preschool if, instead of Miss Michelle trying for the nth time to settle an argument after one gang of kids took over the sandcastle from another gang and made architectural improvements, Mr. Kyle were to assert authority and sort the gangs out the old-fashioned way. Allow me to let my imagination flow a bit, now: maybe Kyle even has a beard...

What I actually mean to say is, an astonishing number of young men are not personally acquainted with their penises, and quite possibly other aspects of their masculinity as well. Somehow they find their way to my practice—not always voluntarily, of course. Unfortunately, from a developmental psychological standpoint, I can't make up for the destruction of the miniature medieval castle in the sandpit. I can, however, encourage the man lying firmly on his hands and chatting about the beaches of Bora Bora to risk opening his eyes to take a look at his glans glowing in the midday sun. I can point out to him that pulling back his foreskin is not an act of violence. Beneath the Bora Bora sun, he hadn't even noticed I'd done it. I've had patients who've broken out in a cold sweat at the first sight of the blank tip of their penises, almost as if I'd shown them pictures of gunshot wounds or an open fibular fracture. Their personal relationship to their own sexual organs up until then must have been along the lines of "Don't look, don't touch." But the penis is, as an organ of reproduction, of vital importance to the continuation of our species, which is why the dear Lord, on creating us men, took great care to encourage us to look after our crown jewels. Physical sensitivity is the gauge given to us by evolution, letting us know that what we're dealing with is an extremely important organ—*see* eyes; *see* testicles. If, in the course of your sexual development, you don't follow the right path and really get to know your dick, you will probably, sooner or later, land on the urologist's couch. Sometimes a sexual therapist's couch, but more on that later.

Returning to the car comparison, after the initial shock I invite the patient for a short test drive. What actually happens when you touch the glans with your index finger? Is that really lava sticking to your fingertips? Does the foreskin tear like a stamp when you peel it back beyond the glans? Often the patient's first approaches to his pride and joy are similar to the first attempts at driving a stick shift in a parking lot—first the gears jam, then too little acceleration and the motor stalls. A man's first attempts at pulling back the foreskin are similarly doomed. My tip for getting to know your penis better: open a bottle of wine (maybe a nice Australian red), fill the bathtub with water (not too hot), and both of you hop in—you and your penis, that is—together with your favorite bath soak.

"Mine's Not That Long, but at Least It's Really Thin!"

"IS IT ACTUALLY normal size?" This is the big question men have. But already here it gets a bit tricky. What *is* a normal-size penis? There are, in fact, statistics that are just as informative as saying "Many men drive Camrys." To follow this riff: if most men's penises are Camrys, a few unfortunate men drive Smart cars and a few lucky ones are sitting in Chevy Tahoes. But, as in real life, many men who drive Camrys, not to mention the Smart car drivers, would love to have a bit more horsepower.

When erect, the Camrys of penises are, according to scientific research, 5 to 6 inches long (12 to 15 centimeters). This is the case no matter where in the world the measurements are taken. Italy, Namibia, and Norway are equally likely to have members of the "long schlong squad" (to quote my colleague M.T. from the Charité, Berlin) who could drive off a pack of wolves by wielding their manhood. To put those numbers in perspective, an average golden hamster (*Mesocricetus auratus*) measures 5 inches (12 centimeters) without its tail. Six inches (15 centimeters) is roughly what you get when you re-create the Facebook "like" symbol at home by placing your fist on a table and measuring to the tip of your thumbnail. And 80 percent of all men are somewhere between a common hamster and a "like," 10 percent above (thumbs up), 10 percent below (thumbs down).

Interestingly, the circumference of a Camry penis is also 5 inches (12 centimeters), so you don't have too much to memorize. Using some high school math, we can quickly calculate the diameter—that's right, somewhere around the 1½ inch (4-centimeter) mark. Now we have the normal penis size as stated in textbooks—erect, of course.

To sum up:

Length: 5–6 inches

Diameter: 1.4 inches

Circumference: 5 inches

By the way, you can also measure the penis in its flaccid state. The erectile tissues are, to a certain degree, flexible reservoirs, able to stretch under pressure. You can stretch and pull a limp willy, and the measurement you arrive at shouldn't differ too much from that of a fully aroused penis.

Patients regularly come to me complaining about driving a Camry. Tahoe drivers are a rare sight in my practice. Men mostly come in on a sexual peace mission, meaning that the penis's "active" length cannot be calculated to the inch. That leaves me with three ways of measuring. Option 1: I pull and stretch the Camry as described above. Option 2: I fetch the previously mentioned silicone breast from the drawer and leave the patient alone with it for a couple of minutes. Option 3: the patient trusts my powers of judgment (after I point out that I have inspected some fifteen penises a day for fifteen years) without the peacock having to display its plumage. Whatever the option, 80 percent of the time we end up within the predicted range—namely, Camry class.

Very rarely, the diagnosis is micropenis—when the erect penis measures less than 2¾ inches (7 centimeters). Several possibilities for such findings should be pursued diagnostically. Often the cause is hormonal irregularities arising from inherited disorders of the pituitary glands. Mutations of the X chromosome, also congenital, are less common. In addition to the real micropenis, there are other circumstances when the penis fails to reach the magical 5-inch mark. These include the buried penis (also called the concealed or inconspicuous penis), the webbed penis, and the trapped penis. In all these forms, the penis—or, rather, the penile shaft—is normal sized but covered by tissue so that it doesn't appear in its full splendor. Surgery, in these cases, helps to make a swan out of an ugly duckling. These diagnoses, however, are extremely rare, and anyway, a swan is only a swan in the eye of the beholder.

So mostly we're dealing with Camrys. The Camry is inspected and measured and we give it its name, but the driver is clearly unhappy with his vehicle. So what now? A new car? That will be difficult.

Let's begin with the medical approach. Basically, a normal penis is not really meant to be lengthened. It doesn't even want to be. There are, however, devices that can keep the cavernous body under constant pressure for weeks and months. Yes, it is basically possible to extend the penile shaft this way. One technology is similar to the balloon-like implants used in transplant medicine. For transplants, the balloons are placed beneath the stomach skin and over time are filled with increasing amounts of liquid so that the skin is stretched. Through the months a kind of skin bag appears above the inflated area. Facial burns can be covered with this surplus skin, or other serious lesions treated. A similar procedure is used nowadays for breast implants. If you wish to extend your penis nonstop over weeks and months this way, I wish you the best of luck. The device looks something like a steel horse harness. Maybe before you start you should think of a few good answers for when your friends and colleagues ask why you're walking around with a hamster cage in your pants.

Then there are vacuum pumps, which can be purchased from all kinds of websites and sex shops. Certainly, these pumps have their relevance in advanced treatment stages of erectile dysfunction. Apart from that, they're useful in reducing postoperative scarring after surgical interventions on the penis. Unfortunately, however, the idea that you can pimp up your Camry with these devices is nonsense. I would also strongly advise against the use of various miracle cures, be they powder, tablet, or magic potion. They just won't work, any more than taking a pill to make your little finger longer. What they will change, however, is the amount of cash in your wallet. We also see DIY regulars who want to take matters into their own hands. Let me tell you—silicone, polyurethane foam, and plastic rulers do not belong under penis skin and are not designed for tinkering with penis length. Regardless of how dissatisfied you are with the size of your johnson, I strongly advise against a visit to the hardware store.

One patient, however, held a different opinion. He had the brilliant idea that if thousands of women can increase the size of their breasts with silicone, then a similar process should work with his penis. No sooner said than done— with one major change in the program. On the spur of the moment in the hardware store, the patient opted for a tube of polyurethane foam from the next shelf over. At home, after a number of shots of hard liquor, he disinfected the tip of a vegetable knife with vinegar to take care of the necessary hygiene. According to the young hardware store shopper who now was lying in the ER with a statue-like object sticking out of his pants, the first cut on the back of his penis was "extremely painful."

"I can well believe that," I replied, marveling at the modern work of art that only vaguely resembled a penis. After the artist had bored a sizable hole in the skin of his penis, allowing a view of his penis shaft, he had poked the foam tube's plastic nozzle into the bleeding hole and squeezed. You know the fairground balloon twisters who create little poodles, hats, and swords? It must have looked something like that as the man pumped a full load of polyurethane foam into his penis. Okay, foam was not perhaps a good choice. But the results *could* be described as impressive.

The amateur artist was able to marvel at his work for a couple of days, and then the first areas of skin began to die off. What we were able to rescue of his penis resembled another product found in hardware stores: a little rubber doorstop.

Years ago I attended a European Congress of Andrology in Madrid. There a Romanian colleague presented a study: he had doubled the length of a penis using body parts from a corpse—somewhat grotesque for my tastes. Frankenstein's monster immediately sprang to mind, and I looked for the screws. We were not informed whether the penis actually worked, but at least it didn't die.

So the penis is difficult to enlarge. If, however, you really feel the need to do so, it can be made broader without taking too many undue risks. Various biological materials can be injected under the outer skin and spread around to increase circumference. Whether sensitivity to touch remains at the desired level? I have no idea. Whether, over time, the injected material calcifies or reshapes other parts of the body? No idea. And how did we put it during residency when we were making fun of ourselves? "Mine's not that long, but at least it's really thin!"

Normally, a man's penis cannot be big enough. In some ways this is like the size of the fish caught by the fraternity of anglers. But I discovered during my first operation at the university hospital of Cologne that the size issue can, sometimes, be the other way around. "Suspected penile carcinoma" was written on the operation plan; my name followed in the column "Surgeon." In carcinoma cases, depending on the particulars of the prior diagnostic findings, a sample is taken from the infected area for a final biopsy analysis under the microscope. Sometimes a generous amount of tissue is removed; occasionally emasculation—off with everything!—is necessary. Before the cancerous growth is cut out with sharp steel, as with all operations, the surgeon should appraise the situation first hand. So, in a free minute, I rushed to the patient's room to introduce myself as his trusty surgeon and took the opportunity to ask him to undress. First he peeled off his shirt, and my first glimpse was of two glistening nipple rings. *Goodness gracious!* I thought. *Is that really necessary, at your age?* I then looked the man in the face and a little more closely: age about fifty, the twenty earrings and nose piercings on both sides of the face a matter of taste. The man's stomach was decorated with a large tattoo in Maori style. I was already curious about the southern regions, below the belt. And I wasn't disappointed! Once the gentleman had discarded his pants, a huge something-or-other emerged from his scrotum—big as a soccer ball, unwrinkled, and red as a baboon's bum. But on closer inspection, I was unable to discover anything that supported the diagnosis for the planned operation, not even a penis. I looked at the gentleman. He looked at me. We both looked at his scrotum—in silence. Finally, I asked, "Where is your penis?"

"Somewhere in there," he replied, looking south with interest. And indeed, on the front of his soccer ball could be seen a slit that on further inspection led deeper.

"What happened?" I inquired with genuine curiosity.

"One day I simply lost interest in my dick. I didn't want to cut it off, so I just tried to inject it away—silicone straight into my ballsack. That was a couple of years ago. One week ago it began to bleed, so I went to my doctor, and he sent me to you."

"Yeah, okay," I said. "Your doctor did the right thing. But why did you want to make your penis disappear?"

Then he told me about some of his sexual problems, the disappointments in his love life and other relationship dramas, and that after a few weeks he bought silicone at the hardware store and syringes at the drug store and started trials to rid himself of the source of all evil. On closer inspection, I found that the whole thing felt like a monster meatball, and I didn't have the faintest idea where to find a penis in this pile of tissue. My very first case—what an introduction to surgery! The next day we got down to business and carefully burrowed around in the mighty soccer ball. Eventually, from the depths of the sack, my surgical scissors knocked against something and there came a sound like a small bell. Lo and behold, after further mining, the glans saw the light of day, pierced lengthwise and crosswise by metal bars with balls screwed on to stop them slipping out. For years this maltreated glans had been sunk in darkness, and now it lay infected and bleeding in front of us. A little bit more excavation and I sewed the penis onto the skin above the scrotum. It wasn't a pretty sight, but still, better than cancer.

SO WHAT DO we do with a Camry that doesn't want to be a Camry? The first premise at our practice is that if someone comes to us, it's because they have a problem, so we take them seriously. And I believe that's the right approach. Time and again patients tell me about seeing other doctors, and the lack of empathy astonishes me. Having too small a penis is no metastasized renal cell cancer and doesn't require a robot-assisted prostate operation, but even so, nobody chooses an affliction just for fun. Every man wants his trusted doctor to listen to what he says without having to hear stupid responses.

In my consulting room I have a small reproduction of an old Michelangelo statue; his name, I think, is David. For centuries, despite his small penis, David has been a symbol of beauty and masculinity. When I'm discussing diagnostic findings, David often finds his way to the middle of my desk to counter the giants. It's often younger men who are dissatisfied with their penis length. Maybe I'm sticking out my neck here, but I can imagine that the gentlemen in question don't look for comparisons in their gym shower but rather visit porn sites, where the "long schlong squad" is occupationally at home. Jockeys are small, basketball players big—know what I mean? Here too it can sometimes be helpful to send the patient to the changerooms at the local pool just to put things in an anatomical perspective before, grief-stricken, he comes up with some absurd plan of action.

Finally, I would like to note two effective alternatives that, when necessary—although they don't actually extend the penis—make it *seem* a lot longer. On examining patients who think their penises are too small, I find that it's very often not the penis that is too small but everything around it that is too big. Try sticking a matchstick in a pea; now try sticking one in a melon. If puppy fat hasn't completely vanished or middle age is already spreading, the suprapubic fat deposits, in the ominous area of the pubic zone below the belt, are often pronounced. The penis almost completely disappears in fatty tissues. During examination, the penile shaft can be exposed all the way to the pelvic ring simply by shifting the fatty tissues aside. If the situation allows the patient to help, the results are even more emphatic. By the way, while we're here, one interesting scientific study has found that if you lose just a bit over 20 pounds (10 kilograms), the penis is already almost an inch longer!

Another possible way to make the penis seem larger is a simple operation. The place where the penis pokes out of the body is by no means its end. The corpus cavernosum runs behind the pelvic bone deep into the body. With it, the penis is anchored deep, like a flagpole in the ground, and can withstand even the roughest of storms. At the pelvic bone, the penile shaft is held in place by two short ligaments. These enable the erect penis to stand straight, which greatly simplifies penetration of the corresponding part of the female anatomy. If you cut through these ligaments, the penis will hang down out of the body by a couple of inches. An erection is still possible, but the erect penis will just dangle down like a cane on a senior's arm. Every man must decide for himself whether this would be beneficial to his libido.

Only once have I had a patient complain about having an oversized member. On examining him, I understood what he meant. Sex with his partner was simply impossible, and up to then only one woman had been able to absorb his anatomy. But, once again, there are no miracle pills or routine operations we can offer with a clear conscience. I've read in scientific journals about penile reduction surgery, in which an incision is made along the length of the penis and cakelike wedges are cut out of each side of the penile shaft. The penis is then collapsed like an accordion and sewn together. It didn't sound particularly enticing, and conjures up an image of an empty hotdog bun.

It sometimes feels as if I've seen 10,000 penises over the course of my career, and I can remember just one or two that could aptly be described as Olympic. One retired professor we were supposed to perform a cystoscopy on (visually examining the interior of the bladder and urethra) had a penis of more modest dimensions, but the catheter was too short to reach the bladder. Ultimately, instead of using the normal cystoscope we had to use a urethroscope, which is twice as long and something we usually use for examining kidneys. Then there was the high-profile American actor who happened to be in Berlin when kidney stones started causing havoc. I had the honor of placing double J stents to relieve him of his renal colic. The anesthetist, fascinated, could only gush, "What a monster!" while measuring the man's penis against his forearm.

The record holders in the penis Olympics carry around organs over 12 inches (30 centimeters) long. These include both the often-mentioned "blood penises" and the rather ugly-sounding "flesh penises." Initially, a blood penis seems to be rather small; it reaches its extreme dimensions only when aroused. Putting it metaphorically, you could say that this is an efficient size adaptation, like an angler's telescopic fishing rods or leporello binding. Leporello binding is an ingenious way of folding pages—for instance, train schedules where you can follow your route through the countryside by unfolding the concertina-like pages. The name is derived from Don Giovanni's servant in the opera of the same name. In the story, Leporello has to compile a list of his master's pan-European love affairs on this sort of sheet for posterity. In the legendary aria "Madamina, il catalogo è questo," he sings of the thousand and three conquests of Mozart's hero in Spain alone—but that is another matter.

The flesh penis, on the other hand, impresses in its splendor even when flaccid. Optimists might think of it as a bird of paradise; pessimists are more likely to compare it to an unrentable vacation home. The elasticity of the tunica albuginea dictates whether what you're looking at is a blood penis or a flesh penis. *Tunica albuginea* is the medical term for the fibrous covering of the cavernous body that, when in use, fills with blood and, with increasing pressure, develops a full capacity for copulation. You can measure the penis length without the sexually driven increase in blood flow if you pull and stretch the penis long enough. One of my colleagues at the Charité once coined the wonderful term "double schlong" for blood and flesh penises.

Why Is the Penis a Penis?

WHY IS A penis a penis, or, to put it another way, how does this quirk of nature actually work? I have vague memories from my wild and impulsive youth of, flashing through my mind, highly philosophical thoughts—unusual for the time—concerning the diversity of the penis. I was at a party, and the consumption of numerous beers had necessitated a visit to the john. It wasn't a particularly attractive room;

a florist's smells better. Behind a locked door I heard the staccato moans typical of two people becoming physically acquainted with each other. So there I stood at the urinal, not particularly impressed with my own mundane business. The austere interior design and the olfactory sensations of the liaison of urine and toilet stalls merely served to underline my impression. Not six feet away, however, behind a locked door, a fellow male was using the same organ system as me. But while he was conducting *his* business, his serotonin levels were probably going through the roof. The love of his life had stolen his heart, and he would probably be talking about this experience for the next ten years—what am I saying: his whole life. Well, okay, I'm relating this experience again after twenty years, but I didn't realize then that I would be writing an infotainment book on urology.

One organ, two functions. Whether we like it or not, we have to cope with this penile diversity. To begin with, I'd like to concentrate on the interpersonal aspects of this one-eyed Dumbledore. Let's take a look at the anatomy.

The penis consists of three cavernous bodies, two of which are actually meant for sex. They fill with blood when necessary, swell up, and, at times, build up enormous pressure. The result is a magnificent erection.

The urethra is embedded in the third cavernous body. During an erection, this cavernous body also fills with blood (which is why you can't pee with morning wood), but it's not crucial for intercourse. This third cavernous body ends at the tip of the glans.

The erection is, on the face of it, a simple thing. Blood streams in, the body expands, pressure rises. But considering

that we don't necessarily want an erection when we're standing in front of the cheese counter in the local supermarket on
a Saturday, and considering how difficult it is to return to an
operational temperature, perhaps there's a somewhat more
subtle regulation hiding in there somewhere.

Why don't we always walk around with an erection if the
penis, like all other organs, has a continuous supply of blood
running through it? The blame—thank goodness—lies with
the sympathetic nervous system (SNS), which, from its base
in the upper spinal column, looks after the genital region.
The SNS suppresses the erection in all everyday situations
by reducing its diameter and restricting the flow of blood to
the blood vessels that cause an erection. When we see our
sweetheart—that person from the class next door or that
model on the magazine stand—a sexual impulse is sent to
the brain and the parasympathetic nervous system (PSNS)
takes over. A touch, smell, or even a thought is sufficient
to release mediators like nitrogen monoxide or acetylcho-
line and thus ban the sympathetic nervous system from the
brain stem, enabling the PSNS from the lower spinal cord to
give the order "open up the sluices" to the arteries feeding
the cavernous body. Through the increased flow of blood
from the arteries the cavernous body tissues absorb blood
like a dry sponge, fill up, and swell. So much blood can be
pumped into the penile shaft that the pressure in the penis
significantly exceeds normal blood pressure levels. With
a systolic blood pressure of 500 mm Hg, 90 percent of
the population would be at the receiving end of a massive
cerebral hemorrhage. If the penis becomes too full of blood,
then the veins that allow the blood to flow back to the body

are forced to the outer peripheral areas of the penis. The erection is an erection thanks to the PSNS and the open arteries. After an orgasm, the SNS is again called for, the feeding blood vessels become narrower, the influx of blood reduces, the veins in the penile shaft refill with blood, and the erection diminishes.

The Glans

THE GLANS, ALSO called the head of the penis, is covered by the foreskin. The outer part of the prepuce, as specialists call it, is just an extension of the skin on the penile shaft (so it consists of normal skin) and is pretty robust. The inner portion, shimmering and shiny when the foreskin is drawn back, is coated in a mucous membrane and is considerably more sensitive. Here too are found Meissner's corpuscles, thousands of tiny alarm systems that are activated at the slightest touch, reacting like a bucketful of gas in a furnace. This makes the foreskin one of the most sensitive parts of the male body.

For this reason you should consider very carefully if and when the foreskin should be removed, whether for cosmetic or other reasons. With a circumcision, you lose an awful lot of nerve endings that are collectively connected to a huge amount of pleasure and fun. During my time as an intern, there was an ancient attending physician who was well known throughout the hospital for his pithy remarks. In the corridor outside the operating theater, a surgeon addressed him about the advanced age of a patient who was being prepared for a circumcision. "I don't understand it either," muttered the urologist. "Wanking just won't be fun anymore." Ah, urologists—sophisticated as ever.

The foreskin continues with the frenulum, the elastic band of tissue under the glans. If the inner sheath of the foreskin is sensitive, then the frenulum is the king of all sensitive areas. The frenulum is, by design, a little on the short side, so that during an erection and the swelling of the glans there is a pull on the band. This makes it even more sensitive, as it activates Meissner's corpuscles.

Textbooks often mention that the foreskin keeps the glans tender and moist, protecting it from injury, grime, damaging environmental impact, drying out, and loss of sensitivity. Fat chance! In my practice, there's little evidence of the foreskin's goody-goody role. Patients normally come to show me their foreskin when there are signs of redness, irritation, inflammation, tearing, or some other form of injury. Sometimes the foreskin is simply too narrow—a condition called *phimosis*, when, in a flaccid state, the foreskin can't be drawn back over the glans. True phimosis is in fact pretty unusual. Many men have problems with the foreskin on erection before sexual intercourse. Either the foreskin is too narrow and tears slightly, leading to inflammation—and, of course, pain—or patients are suffering from what specialists term *paraphimosis*, when the foreskin becomes trapped behind the glans and doesn't return to its former position, for which we advise a rapid solution. The trapped foreskin can swell, increasingly constricting the flow of blood to both the foreskin and the penis. In extreme cases, this can lead to a number of issues from tissue necrosis to major surgery. However, by no means does every foreskin that becomes trapped behind the glans have to be removed. Sometimes lubricants can help the foreskin slip back in position.

Incidentally, extended foreplay with one's partner can have a similarly positive effect, lubricating all the body parts involved. If the (fore)skin is generally dry, regular use of a moisturizing lotion can make the skin more elastic and a bit more resistant to minor tears.

If the foreskin has become constricted owing to the formation of lesions after recurrent inflammation, the transformations can be reversed, at least in the early stages. In such cases I recommend high doses of arginine, an amino acid that is also used in treating erectile dysfunction. Arginine encourages the growth of new blood vessels. Scarring on the foreskin causes the smallest blood vessels to die off so that the tissue becomes increasingly less elastic and slowly shrinks. In some cases the situation can be reversed with improved circulation, making surgery unnecessary. Mild cortisone creams can also be used as a supplemental measure. In exceptional cases, if these forms of treatment prove to be insufficient in curing recurrent or chronic foreskin inflammations, an immunosuppressant ointment, such as tacrolimus, can be tried.

If all these strategies fail, the decision whether to circumcise should be made fast. Advanced inflammation makes it difficult to maintain the standards of hygiene that this part of the body needs, and the spread of scarring to the frenulum means less favorable conditions for good surgical results.

My Foreskin Is Stuck on My Frenulum!

THE FRENULUM IS an elastic band of tissue that connects the foreskin to the glans. It is, as mentioned earlier, a proverbial bundle of nerves. Here you will find nerve fibers careering around like racing cars at Le Mans. And quite rightly so, because that way there's a fixed point you can rely on during sex.

But the anchoring tissue is no ship's rope. Rather, it's a tender mucosa band, like that found beneath the tongue, on the upper and lower lip, the clitoris, and parts of the rectal suspensory apparatus. If you bear in mind that during sexual intercourse a male of medium weight—165 pounds (75 kilograms)—is moving perpendicularly toward the center of the earth, it's hardly surprising that without enough vaginal lubrication, these fickle tissues will show signs of wear and tear. Lubrication is the amount of vaginal moisture present, and it determines, along with the partner's arousal through foreplay, the lube level. The fact that "lube level" here sounds a bit disrespectful has a not completely insignificant background: regardless of the male anatomy, for many women any sort of foreplay is, of course, an important part of a satisfactory sex life. Where sex is concerned, men tend to be like gas stoves: switched on and immediately hot. Women often behave more like older electric stoves: they need some time until the temperature is right. Additionally, the state of lubrication often depends on the amount of time spent on foreplay. And now, for everyone who still hasn't grasped it: the longer and more intense the foreplay, the lower the risk that the man will damage his frenulum.

What happens when, despite plenty of mutual attention, the guitar strings of the penis become unduly strained and break, with a high-pitched ping? Running through the frenulum along with the neural race track is the arteria frenularis. What was that from high school biology about arteries and veins? Veins transport used, low-oxygen blood at relatively low pressure back to the heart, from where the blood is pumped to the lungs to be enriched with oxygen. Blood from vein wounds is dark because of the low oxygen content, and it trickles slowly from the wound because of the low pressure. Arteries are governed by considerably higher pressure. A damaged artery will spurt much more blood from the wound, blood that is a lighter red. This is why, in general, arteries are deeper inside the body: to protect against greater loss of blood. The trouble is that for the frenulum, roughly one-half of one-tenth of an inch thick (1 millimeter), there is no "deep," making the frenulum the Achilles heel of arterial blood supply. And regardless that a mosquito can pee with more force than the arteria frenularis can pump blood, a rip in the frenulum is very painful and can cause an almighty mess in the bedroom—a few scary moments are guaranteed for those concerned. Even more annoyingly, the open wounds often become inflamed. After all, the vaginal tract is not exactly a sterile environment ... but more of that later. It can take a few weeks for the wound to heal. Occasionally, young males in the springtime of their sexual creativity experience what it means to walk around with a ripped frenulum. It's difficult to be abstinent when the end-of-term party beckons, but unfortunately, it's sometimes the only option. Those without strong resolve are condemned to almost endless repetition of this cycle. The problem arises from the disrupted and delayed healing process: the longer it takes, the more scarring in the injured area, and the more scar tissues, the more the shrinkage to the frenulum in the scarred region. The more the frenulum shrinks, the more the tension at the next attempt at sexual intercourse, and the greater the tension, the more likely the frenulum is to rip again. It's a urological mother of all vicious circles.

So, what to do if the frenulum tears? First of all, remain calm. When the night of cozy togetherness ends abruptly and a visit to the local emergency unit beckons, it all seems very dramatic, but basically nothing has happened that has seriously endangered anything. You'll lose more blood from an accident with a potato peeler, and no one has died from that.

Normally, you can halt the bleeding in half an hour by grabbing the nearest tissue, or anything else reasonably sterile within reach, and pressing it to the wound. The diameter of the artery is so small that this will stop the flow of blood. It's enough then to take a peek the next morning and marvel at the intactness of your pride and joy. That said, you should look more carefully at the wound. If you're lucky, the frenulum will have torn right through to the penile trunk. I know—most people don't like the sound of that. The point is that we urologists would do little else during an operation. Okay, you have a local anesthetic, in sterile conditions, and have to take a few cosmetic considerations into account, and then the frenulum is sliced with a scalpel down to the trunk of the penis. One clear disadvantage of surgery is that if the frenulum is severed, it is then, for cosmetic reasons, removed completely. This means stitches, and it can take up to a month for the stitches to dissolve. Any form of sexual intercourse should be avoided during this time, as it could lead to further bleeding or infection. After a hot-blooded tear and the subsequent pressure bandage, on the other hand, the penis only has to be confined to quarters for a couple of days, provided an infection can be avoided. This isn't rocket science: a chamomile bath, a little healing ointment, and for a few days mobilizing the poor patient when you pee.

If the frenulum isn't totally severed, you can reckon with the formation of scar tissues and contraction, in the above-described causal chain. In this case, early local application of cortisone cream is advisable, in order to keep the scarring as minimal as possible. Take things easy until the wound has completely healed. If the frenulum continues to tear, then sooner or later, an operation will be unavoidable. And the more scarring to the frenulum, the more difficult it will be for the operation to turn out well.

Bumps and Spots

PEARLY PENILE PAPULES

Pearly penile papules is the term given to tiny protuberances, or bumps—sometimes more, sometimes less visible—that form on the lower ridge of the glans. Sometimes you need a magnifying glass to see them. In rare cases, however, these tiny things can be as big as a few hundredths of an inch, which *can* cause cosmetic problems. But the important point is that there's nothing that you can—or, rather, should—do about them. Firstly, *hirsuties papillaris*, as they're known to the initiated, are by no means harmful. They have absolutely no pathological significance, and on the danger scale are on par with receding hairlines and freckles. Furthermore, I have never known pearly penile papules to become symptomatic, apart from cosmetically. Here too they're on par with hair color or a gap in your front teeth. If you did want to remove the tiny papules, it would have to be through surgery—there are no pills or lotions that can do the trick. It *is* theoretically conceivable to remove them with a scalpel or laser, but because the ridge of the glans is incredibly well supplied with blood, such an operation would cause both an awful mess and, with biblical certainty, serious scarring to the glans.

A RED SPOT IS A RED SPOT IS A RED SPOT

On the day that the Soviet red star was removed from the humongous parliamentary building in Budapest, I was by chance visiting the city on the Danube. The cab driver obviously couldn't believe his eyes—stopped in the middle of the road as if he had seen a jovial Captain Kirk waving at him from the passenger seat of the USS *Enterprise* above the hill behind the Hotel Gellért.

Sometimes, but only very seldom, I wish that not only would the red star vanish into thin air but so would the red spot. For urologists, this would be as historic as the removal of the Communist emblem was for my cab driver.

Our fraternity and our afflicted patients describe the red spot the same: a red spot. Likes to sit on the glans, quite happy on the foreskin. Sometimes about a tenth of an inch (2 to 3 millimeters), but preferably invisible! As I've said, I try to empathize equally with every patient, regardless of whether we are talking about renal cancer, infertility, or a foreskin infection. When someone says, "I had a red spot somewhere on my glans that vanished three weeks ago, but I thought, 'Better safe than sorry,'" of course I take a look and offer my patient advice. If, however, the gentleman has registered in my clinic as an emergency case and expects to cut in line ahead of a renal colic patient or someone with a recently discovered testicular cancer in our emergency consulting time slot, then he'd better be prepared for a slightly longer wait.

Men! Don't be stupid! A red spot on your glans is, in the majority of cases, the same as a red spot on your face: a minor inflammation. Others would call it a pimple. If you think about how often the pink-helmeted warrior of love comes into contact with bacteria while being used sometimes more, sometimes less tenderly, it's only to be expected that every now and then the surface of the glans will acquire a slight redness. The inflammation normally vanishes within a few days. But here too, the better the lubrication, the fewer microscopic injuries can be expected on the skin of the glans and the more difficult it will be for bacteria to get beneath the skin and trigger an inflammation.

Sexually Transmitted Diseases

GENITAL WARTS

Genital warts are no source of happiness for those concerned, and even well-versed laypeople find their proper names pretty difficult to enunciate. They are called *condylomata acuminata* or *mollusca contagiosa*, and sound rather like grand dames of Argentinian tango. Apart from the hint of South American flair, there is little else to make them attractive. These finger- or lentil-shaped warts appear from the waistline down, just where they're least wanted—on the penis, scrotum, foreskin, glans, inner upper thigh, and pubic zone. These are nice fertile areas, including for the human papillomavirus (HPV) and *Molluscipoxvirus* (a member of the Poxviridae family), as they swarm like a stag party at a bar during happy hour and start causing annoying, itchy irritation.

The transformation is initially hardly visible, so much so that even I can't be certain whether they're mini genital warts and thus the beginning of a long shared journey or simply everyday gland follicles that have become slightly inflamed after sloppy genital shaving, or, to put it another way, just pimples. The other end of the scale is, like the famous Richter scale, open-ended. Condylomata can grow not only to the size of lentils or rice but to the size of cherries. By then most patients are considering whether a visit to their urologist might be a good option. *Buschke-Löwenstein tumor* is the name given to a kind of exploding condyloma the size, shape, and weight of which make it very much resemble a cauliflower, although the green and white are replaced by gray and flesh tones.

These viruses are transmitted via sex, but sexual intercourse as such doesn't have to have occurred. Intensive mutual petting is enough to transport HPV or the virus *Molluscum contagiosum* from A to B. Even more ominous, condoms don't protect against transmission. Most of the time the warts first appear in the pubic bone area. If you want to ensure that the infection isn't transferred, you had better place a heavy shopping bag—or better still, a tarp—between you and your partner. This, however, does tend to lose you points on the romantic front, which is why it is often dismissed as a solution when partners are first getting to know one another.

Being the carrier of a virus doesn't mean you're ill. Pathologically, the first sign that you're a carrier is the already described skin transformation. Whether warts appear, however, depends on your immunity. You can quite comfortably and happily live with your viral lodgers without even noticing them. But if your immune system begins to falter—for instance, because of a severe cold, prolonged stress, or a weekend of heavy partying—these things pop up out of nowhere. The heavier the load on the immune system, the more impressive the skin manifestations. I've had patients who after a night on the town wake up not only with a monumental hangover but also with an army of forty-plus warts presenting arms. (While we're on the subject of sex and celebrations, the annual peak in the condylomata season in Cologne happens to be shortly after our annual carnival.)

If you're really fortunate, the virus that causes the un-welcome genital warts strays to the urethra and then disappears down the urinal, though in the Charité I once had a patient who had a handful of plum-sized condylomata in the bladder—not a pretty sight.

Another piece of good news is that the warts usually stay small and have more of a cosmetic effect than a serious disease-causing one. There is, of course, a rider: usually is not always. The real problem with HPV infections is that the family of the human papillomavirus is a large one: there are more than 140 known types of human papillomaviruses. And as in all extended families, one or another uncle or great-niece likes to misbehave. So it is with HPV16, HPV18, and HPV23, which can cause cancer. For men, this is cancer of his pride and joy: penile cancer. Luckily, penile cancer is extremely rare. For women, unfortunately, the prospects are worse: the high-risk human papillomaviruses cause 95 percent of cervical cancer cases. There is now a vaccine against a number of the carcinogenic HPV family members. However, vaccination is recommended *before* sexual intercourse has taken place. For many who are already virus carriers, then, it's probably ineffective, and it will be decades before an immunization effect similar to, say, tetanus can be achieved. Moreover, the cost of the vaccination in many places is covered by insurance only for girls; boys—or rather, their parents—have to pay out of pocket.

It is possible to carry out tests to discover whether a man is an HPV carrier, and every week I'm visited by worried men. However, I recommend against the test for most people for the following reasons: First, the tests don't seem to me to be 100 percent reliable. Every now and then a patient with histologically documented condylomata obtains an HPV-negative reading from the serum tests—which can't possibly be accurate. We've tried a test in which we scrub away at the condylomata, something like using a wire brush, to get material to compare and contrast with existing HPV strains, but here too we sometimes get misleading results.

Second, there's no cure for HPVs that are already circulating in the bloodstream. There is no targeted therapy, unlike, for instance, for herpes viruses. Research will have to show whether, one day, vaccination against HPV will cushion the spread of the disease. For now the only one who can control the beasts already in the system is the patient, or rather, his immune system. To this end, it can definitely be helpful to lead a healthy lifestyle. Alas, in this case, that doesn't mean just "No French fries today": the immune system is interested in a long-term commitment. Should physical activity, stress reduction, and a healthy diet prove insufficient to accomplish this, then maybe a visit to the drug store might help. There are several immune-strengthening combination products available on the market. Besides the various vitamins, trace elements and antioxidants are important. Scientific literature often cites low vitamin D levels as being associated with the pathological course of HPV infections. Given that 80 percent of German men lack sufficient vitamin D, it doesn't surprise me that I see so many patients with condylomata.

Once the condylomata have appeared, the patient has a number of options. Doing nothing at all, which often turns into even more having to be done later, is the worst option.

Every now and then, however, there are instances of spontaneous healing, which tend to point to a reinforced immune system. Condylomata can be dabbed, smeared, and nursed with all kinds of creams, ointments, and tinctures. You may have noticed that I'm no friend of local therapy, treating just the spot. You can often see an improvement, but *just* an improvement, and usually only a temporary one. When the warts have disappeared from one area, they emerge elsewhere—it's rather like corralling a herd of fleas. On top of this, local therapy takes forever: weeks to months of burning sensations on the skin and messy stains on the underpants and sheets. I much prefer sharp steel, in the form of a scalpel, surgical scissors, or curette (a scraping tool). The local anesthetic in the genital area provides little enjoyment, but the operation takes only a few minutes and afterward all the warts really are gone.

Before an operation to remove condylomata, and with it the maximum reduction in the viral load, I recommend some form of immune-supporting treatment from the drug store, to achieve long-lasting end results.

THE UROLOGICAL PETTING ZOO: GONOCOCCI, CHLAMYDIA, UREAPLASMA, TRICHOMONAS

Anyone who has had an infection of his mast knows that it's no fun. Either you end up scratching at the floor tiles in agony while peeing because the morning visit to the toilet suddenly feels as if you are peeing out a bucketful of rusty thumbtacks, or, despite stuffing three rolls of paper towels in your underpants, there are still thick green stains just where you don't want to have them. When it really gets a grip on you, it smells like Monday morning at the fish counter when "Shrimpy" Sherman forgot the weekend swilling-out ritual. That would be the image of a full-blown gonococci infection, or gonorrhea, affectionately known to connoisseurs as "the clap."

Often the only signs of gonorrhea are small amounts of pus seeping out of the urethral opening and an unpleasant burning sensation while peeing. When this is the case in the early stages, the festering early-morning salutation is sometimes referred to as *"bonjour* drops," which by no means should be confused with the small glass of rosé sipped by a loving couple after a late breakfast on their private all-inclusive-holiday deck. Every now and then progression is atypical, and patients feel a slight tweaking along the urethra, from the anus to the scrotum and along the penis. They then ask themselves whether it might have been more sensible last weekend to use a condom. In most of the unspectacular cases, a differential gonorrhea diagnosis is tricky, and it sometimes feels as if it takes up a fifth of my workday.

Besides gonococci, the most common specific pathogens associated with infections of the urethra are chlamydia and mycoplasma. Their symptoms also include discomfort when peeing, albeit without reaching the heights of rusty thumbtacks. Those afflicted by chlamydia or mycoplasma speak of urethral discharges, but these are mostly watery or transparent and not the greenish yellow of nasty old clap. Unfortunately, with the almost limitless topic of urethral discharges, as with most things in life, there is no black and white—or rather, green and yellow—but a whole spectrum, from slightly unpleasant to a feeling that Armageddon is approaching. The best thing about both chlamydia and mycoplasma infections is that they can often be treated successfully with the same combination of antibiotics and, even better, with just a single high-dosage shot. Today you're at the urologist, tomorrow everything's fine.

All this really wouldn't be a problem were it not for the fact that on top of gonococci and chlamydia and all their relations, there are two more groups. Group three describes those patients suffering from nonspecific infections of the urethra. In these cases, pathogens—the nastier relatives—from the family of intestinal bacteria infect the mucous membrane of the urethra with symptoms similar to the specific urethral infections we just talked about. The problem is that under some circumstances, you need very different antibiotics to kill these ones off. In order to come to a conclusive diagnosis, even in unspectacular cases, we have to start a culture to allow the bacteria to multiply in order to discover its first and second name. This takes at least two days, and the afflicted gentleman, who until now has been literally quite willing to sit out his problem ("I thought it would just go away..."), suddenly doesn't want to wait that long.

The fourth group is considerably trickier, as it behaves more deviously. There are symptoms but no inflammation. Here we have to tread very carefully: no inflammation doesn't mean that the patient isn't ill. As I've often said, every complaint has to be taken seriously. Often symptoms can be traced back to psychosomatic roots—the mind influencing the body—even if the patient isn't initially aware of those causes. More about that in the prostate chapter.

I am regularly asked, "And is a urethral infection dangerous?" And from me the crystal-clear answer: "Yes and no!" Often men are just carriers, especially with chlamydia infections, and therein lies the problem. For women as well—including the female partners of male carriers—chlamydia infections are often asymptomatic. However, in many cases chlamydia leaves women infertile. The infection is often based in a woman's fallopian tubes, whereas for men it settles in the urethra. A reaction to the infection causes adhesion and sealing of the fallopian tubes. The egg produced in the ovaries and released during ovulation races like a toboggan down the fallopian tube toward the sperm, which swim up the cervical canal to the uterus. But if the fallopian tubes are sealed, the egg is confronted with a closed door, like traveling Americans standing outside a French supermarket at noon. No bread for toast, no pregnancy. As for men, urethral infections can also put men's family planning on ice. If the little beasts surge on along the urethra toward the prostate and are feeling up to it, they can continue to the vas deferens and on to the seminal colliculus (the outlet where the vas deferens leads to the prostate), eventually reaching the epididymis. The epididymis is something like a barracks for sperm, where the tiny swimmers await their marching orders. Ejaculation means "Charge!" and a couple of million tadpoles head into no-man's-land. However, they can do so only if their path isn't blocked by an infection like chlamydia. If it's blocked, the released egg, which was supposed to have a rendezvous with a colossal army of admirers numbering half the population of Europe, waits alone and neglected in the uterus. How sad, and what a waste!

DO IT—DESPITE THE POX

Syphilis, a.k.a. the pox, has made people's lives a misery for hundreds of years. It predated even the great-grandparents of Alexander Fleming, the man to be credited, in the far distant future, with the discovery of penicillin. The syphilis bacterium, *Treponema pallidum*, is transmitted during unprotected sexual intercourse and, if untreated for years or even decades, leads to problems that include serious brain and nerve damage. Since Fleming began growing cultures in his laboratory petri dishes and, decades later, penicillin could be bought in every drug store, the bacteria has become almost completely extinct. Dr. Condom's latex sheaths did the rest. But for a number of years now, rampant antibiotics-against-everything treatment, condom-free sex, and sex tourism in Asia and Eastern Europe have led to a considerable rise in cases. I recently read an article claiming that the rise was as much as 600 percent. If bacteria were shares, then I'd say hats off. With a few exceptions, however, syphilis is easy and safe to treat. Two jabs of Dr. Fleming's magic potion, left and right in the bum, and hey, presto! The problem, unfortunately, is that by no means all syphilis patients are treated. This is due not least to the fact that diagnosing the disease from its clinical expression is at times difficult and it is often overlooked.

The first sign of a syphilis infection is little more than a red pimple or boil in the genital region. Depending on a person's sexual practices, the infection can also occur in the mouth or rectum. The bump feels hard, which is why it is termed a *hard chancre*, and not to be confused with the similar-looking soft chancre, which is also transmitted during free-for-alls on the mattress but is considerably less harmful. The soft chancre is, true to its name, soft, but compared to its syphilitic counterpart, much more painful when touched. The hard chancre can be accepted or overlooked. Later the tip of the ulceration collapses, leaving a small crater-like impression—the central necrosis. It's something like a tiny red volcano with a gooey crater—not, however, on Hawaii, but in your underpants. The discharged secretion teems with pathogens and is highly infectious.

Once you have sighted a volcano in your underpants and made an appointment with your trusted urologist, keep this appointment! Even if the appointment is three weeks later and the volcano then *seems* to be history. You might not have a volcano, but you're running around with syphilis and it's highly infectious.

Roughly eight weeks after the initial infection, general symptoms begin appearing that are similar to the flu. On top of this in the second phase, skin inflammations sometimes arise for a couple of weeks. These can be slightly moist and are also highly infectious. Some patients notice lymph node swelling that eases off in a couple of weeks. Those lymph nodes are, unfortunately, still extremely infectious.

Sometimes, years later, other manifestations of the disease appear, ones that require considerably more protracted treatment. In this third phase, there is a danger of organ damage and of rubbery nodules, which don't make the disease any prettier. If things go badly, the heart is involved: the rubbery nodules grow in the middle wall layers of the main artery and, with a slight increase in blood pressure, easily burst.

Should you survive all this (apart from a burst aorta, which would be difficult) to become a syphilis oldie, you end up in the fourth stage: neurosyphilis. This phase is characterized by bulbous transformations in the brain and leads to dementia and death.

So: Condoms make a lot of sense, and a small penis pimple that mysteriously disappears should jolt you into a visit to your trusted urologist for a checkup. Even if it is just a red spot.

Warped Willies and Permaboners

WHEN WAS THE last time you closely inspected your penis? Did anything catch your attention? Does your best friend tend to point to the left or right? Does it have a small indentation rather like the waist? Can you feel a lump beneath the skin that you hadn't noticed previously, and does it stretch out when an erection is on the way? These symptoms could be heralding IPP and, potentially, a season ticket to your urologist. IPP—induratio penis plastica, or Peyronie's disease—is a chronic disease of the soft tissue of the penis. The disease is quite common: depending on which studies you read, it can affect up to 8 percent of men. That's almost as frequent as diabetes in the United States, so we're dealing here with an extremely widespread problem.

The typical symptoms of IPP are tactile deformations of the penis, often linked to curving or bending and, in later stages, to a shortening of the penis. The bending or buckling is gradual, but with the progression of the disease, it can reach angles of 90 degrees or more—and sex with a penis the shape of a door handle or fish hook is only possible for acrobats. Furthermore, pain and general erectile dysfunction can occur, which don't make the situation any more pleasant. I have one IPP patient in my practice who has to fall back on morphine to keep the pain reasonably tolerable.

The deformations are excessive lesions to the erectile tissues caused by bending and twisting during sexual intercourse. Why some people are affected and others not remains unclear. The precise reason for penile bending is also unknown. Genetics is one possibility, as patients suffering from this disease share a chromosomal mutation. Typically, though, patients speak of a recent sex mishap in which the penis slipped out and then rammed against the partner's body.

Generally speaking, the disease runs through various phases. During the first, acute phase, which can last a year or more, the symptoms become increasingly stronger, with inflammatory processes in the erectile tissues playing a role. If the symptoms remain unchanged, the stable phase has been reached. Here, calcification can appear in the area of the lesions, which eventually feel somewhat like bones in the penis when touched. Treatment should begin early in the active, inflammatory phase—once the bonelike structures have become established, it will be harder to reach a satisfactory result.

When an IPP patient is first diagnosed, an examination of the penile tissue is carried out in order to discover how far along the disease is. Then an ultrasound examination is essential to eliminate the above-mentioned calcification of the penile lesions. In some cases, hormonal analysis—checking individual metabolic values—is useful to diagnose secondary complications. Photos of the penis are another important diagnostic tool, to measure and track the curvature or indentation of the penile tissue before and during treatment. Patients are naturally not over the moon when I ask them to bring photos of their erect bent penises! Ultimately, however, they see the point when, with the aid of the photos, I measure the precise degree of the curvature with an orthopedic protractor, which enables me to better assess the treatment procedure. On top of this, at the beginning and during treatment, pain levels and quality of life should be monitored.

If the damage has already been done, there remains a whole range of drug therapies. The snag is that the drugs on offer don't always help, sometimes have marked side effects, and are sometimes extremely expensive. If you suspect that you have a case of IPP, you should drop in to your local drug store and ask for high-dosage vitamin E, and ask your physician about where to acquire the energy converter L-carnitine. Both have, in a number of cases, led to an easing of the symptoms. At the same time, try to take it easy on your penis. During sexual intercourse or anything else you or your penis may encounter, make sure no intense shearing forces damage the penile tissues. After all, it was because of the severe buckling effects and microscopic wounds to the tissues that the disease took root in the first place.

It's also helpful for your misshapen friend to get a bit of care and affection in an unerect state. Massage and knead the appropriate areas against the direction of the kink. With this stretching exercise, the lesions and lumpy areas of the penile tissues should loosen up and become more flexible. Inflammation can be reduced with some ibuprofen. If the medication available over the counter doesn't make a fundamental difference, there are prescription options. Unfortunately, their effectiveness is not resounding and the probability that the patient will have more or less bearable stomach problems is considerable.

If nothing fundamentally changes after trying out these tips, or if the condition and symptoms even become worse, a lot can be achieved with extracorporeal shock wave therapy (ESWT). Painful erections, which often end up in psychosomatic erectile dysfunction, can be particularly successfully treated by shock wave therapy.

If the penile curvature is chronic, the only option is corrective surgical intervention. There are two different operative methods to get a bent penis back to its desired upright position. In one, the penile tissue on the opposite side of the lesions is shortened using pinch stitching until the penis is straightened (following either the Essed-Schröder or the Nesbit method). The lesions remain, but the curvature is canceled out by artificial lesions created adjacent to them. The operation is relatively quick and has few risks or postoperative complications. It does, however, result in a shortening of the penis length.

The second, and slightly more elegant, method surgically tackles the root problem—namely, the lesions in the penile tissues. The lesion is split during the operation so that the shortening resolves itself. The defect the operation creates on the penile shaft has to be compensated for with a suitable material, rather like a puncture in a bike tire except instead of air leaking out, it's blood. The snag here is that sometimes the lesions run deep into the tissue or between the two cavernous bodies far into the body, requiring a high degree of surgical expertise during the operation to attain a satisfactory result. There are, however, plenty of hospitals that perform this operation with good results.

PRIAPISM

Priapus, the son of Aphrodite and Dionysus in Greek mythology, obviously didn't suffer from these problems. He is depicted as hung like a horse—although he is only as tall as Tom Cruise. In Greek mythology, Priapus is the god of fertility and is generally shown with a penis that is almost bigger than he is. Priapism is a decidedly delicate and ill-fated diagnosis. The term describes a condition in which the penis remains erect in the absence of sexual stimulation. After a couple of hours, it begins to become extremely painful; after six hours, the penis has had it, and there's a real risk of long-term erectile dysfunction. The venous (oxygen-deficient) blood no longer flows out of the penis to return to the heart for more oxygen, and after a few more hours this causes tissue damage to the cavernous body and massive disruption to the functions of the capillaries. What remains is a compact, small penis that, even with higher rates of blood flow, can no longer swell. The cause of priapism is often congenital blood disease in which the shape of the red corpuscles sometimes transforms bizarrely, impairing the flow properties of the blood. It's also not uncommon for a sexually overindulgent man who, on top of other drugs, has downed an Olympic dose of Viagra to appear rather sheepishly in the ER a few hours later with a colossal erection that will not abate.

During my time at the Charité, I encountered a number of such cases on night duty. I remember my first case pretty clearly. I was called out of bed late at night. The triage nurse was giggling, which I found a bit odd. Somewhat sleepy, I managed to grasp that I had to get down there quickly—it was an emergency. A young man lay in the treatment room under a blanket that resembled a circus tent. His girlfriend was sitting next to him and was just as drunk as he was but in considerably less pain. Of course I had heard and read about priapism, the mother of all urological emergencies, but I hadn't had the pleasure of witnessing it live and in color. I moved the blanket to one side and saw an impressive piece of tackle, which was, typically for priapism, pointing up to the ceiling. A few hours previously the couple had both swallowed hallucinogenic stimulants, and the gentleman had topped it off with 300 milligrams of Viagra. He could have cracked open a bank safe with his rock-hard erection. As always in emergencies I tried to create as serene an impression as possible and disappeared, remarking that I had to get some blood vials. Hastily I began leafing through the red-rimmed emergency pages of my clinical urology handbook. What then happened was one of my first cases of "Urology is a funny old business," to be followed by many more in the coming years.

The diagnosis of the disease required—please fasten your seat belts—broaching the penis with a cannula, a tube, to establish the pH level of the blood. I already had recognized that the dark, almost black color of the blood meant that it must be venous and low in oxygen, but measurement is needed for proper records. So now came what my supervisor, who had been alerted and who knew all the tricks of the trade, called the "vice." Under his supervision, I jabbed a really thick cannula, which he had selected, deep into the penis of the increasingly docile party monster. My fist enclosed the almost movingly piteous patient's member while the end of the cannula, which would have been at home in veterinary medicine (in the large and wild animal department), poked out between my middle and ring fingers. "And now—give it some oomph, Gralla!" the good professor prompted me. The blood squirted in all directions while my mentor tried in vain to catch the black sludge in a kidney dish, but everything landed on my mentor's plump belly. His eyes gleamed. He had obviously enjoyed navigating me through the rocky waters of urological emergency procedures, and I felt as if my father had taught me how to fish. The man and his girlfriend, who had in the meantime chosen to leave the room, were taken to the ward.

Should you happen to be noticed with an inappropriate erection while walking through a Brazilian banana plantation, you have probably been bitten by *Phoneutria nigriventer*, commonly known as the Brazilian wandering spider—an aggressive little beast that jumps at its victims. The bite of this spider causes not only great pain but also an imposing erection verging on priapism, which has guaranteed jobs for a number of men and women in the research branch of pharmacology. In 2015, Brazilian researchers published a study in which they described how they had synthetically produced the active agents of the toxin. Viagra and co. be warned!

two

THE PROSTATE: GOD'S ROGUE ORGAN

W E ALL MAKE mistakes—you, me, Mozart, Babe Ruth, George Clooney, and dear old God. While relaxing on Sunday after, let's face it, a pretty eventful week, something must have happened to really annoy him. Maybe he was bitten by the neighbor's dog, his team lost the tournament, or he was out and about with a few friends and up to mischief. Something was amiss, or on Monday he wouldn't have given us men a prostate.

The prostate is like Timbuktu: everyone has heard of it but nobody knows where it is. Or a catalytic converter—everyone's car (electrics excepted) has got one, but nobody knows how it works. The prostate: an enigma, a legend, a mystery...

The prostate is a small ball of muscle deep under a man's pelvis. God probably buried it so deep because he had a guilty conscience about overburdening his blueprint for humanity with an organ like this one. The prostate lies directly beneath the bladder; the urethra runs right through it. When you go for a pee, you are peeing, as it were, through the prostate. Up to puberty it is roughly the size of a chestnut, and a similar shape—so, slightly heart-shaped. That is its only resemblance to a heart. After puberty, in the course of decades, prostates can reach absurd sizes and make us men's lives hell. And even if the beast *does* remain the size of a chestnut, that's no cause to sound the all-clear sirens. Urological prudence is the better part of valor.

The prostate is a gland, so it produces secretions. The seminal vesicles, a pair of tubular glands the shape and size of a finger, are attached to the prostate like a double backpack, and together with it form a unit. The three are inseparable, like Huey, Dewey, and Louie, or sun, moon, and stars, or hamburgers, ketchup, and mustard. The slimy product of the prostate and its backpack colleague end up in the urethra. But not always—only when you just happen to be having an orgasm. Over 90 percent of the male DNA mix comes from the prostate and vesicles. Less than 10 percent comes from the scrotum and a couple of other production centers. This is why ejaculation after a vasectomy, in which the vas deferens are severed so that sperm can no longer exit, is no different from before the operation.

So what's the point of the prostate and seminal vesicles if sperm comes from somewhere completely different? It's something like a concert: The sperm are the stars of the show and arrive in a stretch limo. All the rest—the amplifiers, the speaker towers, the stage sets, lighting, cables, musicians, catering services, and other bits and pieces—arrive in a fleet of trucks. So no trucks, no concert. And similarly, no prostate and seminal vesicles, no offspring. Pretty much everything that sperm could possibly need on the way to their rendezvous with the ovum is contained in the mush. It's a crazy cocktail of hormones, neurotransmitters, various forms of sugar (as energy donors), zinc, selenium and other salts, proteins, enzymes and amino acids, white blood corpuscles, and even, apparently, traces of gold. There's enough there to accompany even Mariah Carey.

In a nutshell, the prostate makes sperm food. So far, so good. But why does it have to be so complicated? The organ is needed for the creation of offspring. Maybe one child, two, sometimes even three or four. For four children, four ejaculations should suffice. If you happen to have twins, maybe even fewer! An orgasm gives a man maybe five to ten seconds of ecstatic joy; afterward the excitement level returns to normal. In your whole life, you need the prostate for between fifteen to forty seconds for its actual function: procreation. Couldn't something else have been invented, something that doesn't have the potential to get on your nerves for the rest of your life? If you subtract the fun of having four children and the forty seconds, I can hardly think of a better definition of *superfluous*. Agreed, there are plenty of useless things in the world, but a pepper grinder with LED lights doesn't cause bone metastases or kill anyone!

According to the above calculations, the prostate of a man with an average life expectancy of 78 is unnecessary baggage for 77 years, 364 days, 23 hours, 59 minutes, and about 20 seconds. You could even deduct the first 20 years, as very little should go wrong with the organ during that time.

Changes in Bladder Capacity

NORMALLY, PROBLEMS WITH the prostate crop up in the "best years." Mine started just before I was 40, the same sort of age as the patients who appear at my practice with the first flaws in *their* rogue organ. Typical symptoms are changes in bladder capacity—how much they can pee. The frequency increases at first, imperceptibly and then more and more, until "Excuse me, I have to go" becomes a major conversation point. Whereas you used to smile wearily and just put your foot down on the gas pedal till, three exits later, you reached home and could empty your bladder in the confines of your own restroom, now highway service stations are your salvation. Increasingly, underpants noticeably become what they always were unnoticeably—drip catchers. Larger volumes of dripping cause people with prostate problems to sense a real urge to pee again, which leads to a great degree of uncertainty. With increasing age, "staccato" urination becomes an issue: an interrupted flow of small portions of urine, resulting from arbitrary tensing of the pelvic floor and stomach muscles. Eventually sufferers are confronted with nocturia—having to visit the bathroom at night—which, after the third, fourth, or fifth time being dragged out of a sound sleep, is severely disruptive and, according to scientific studies, responsible for increasing the risk of falls and accidents.

The first symptom of change in the prostate is often a weakening of the intensity of the urine stream. On the one hand, this isn't a problem, because you no longer take part in peeing contests against a wall. On the other hand, it's very annoying when the toes of your shoes or even your shoelaces become damp.

Prostate complaints are as varied as a bouquet of flowers, which is why it makes sense to better understand an individual situation by means of specific diagnostics. One important tool is ultrasound, which can help identify the size of the prostate as well as its shape and its position in relation to the bladder. In 90 percent of cases the backside version—an ultrasound rectal probe—is not necessary. The most important data can be gathered by placing the ultrasound transducer on the stomach just below the waistline. This book is called not *Happy from Behind* but *Happy Down Below*! On measuring the prostate's volume, it is often noticeable that symptoms seldom correlate to the size of the organ. There are elderly gentlemen with huge prostates and hardly any complaints; others, however, have smaller glands but are severely plagued. A normal prostate size is difficult to define. The most often detected volumes for 30- to 50-year-olds are around 15 to 30 cc; older patients can have prostates of 40, 50, or even 80 cc. Prostate volumes of 115 cc can be called remarkable. The largest one I have ever measured was 180 cc, a veritable Godzilla.

Size alone, however, is not an indicator that treatment is called for. Ultrasound can also measure residual urine volumes. If, after you pee, considerably more than 200 milliliters of urine remains in the bladder, this could lead to problems in the long term. The frequency of "I have to go" continues to increase as the bladder steadily fills and is more or less continuously under pressure. If the bladder cannot be properly emptied, inflammations will often result. In severe cases, the bladder is so full after peeing that the urine, little by little, accumulates as far back as the kidneys. After years or decades, this can lead to renal failure and trips to the dialysis unit.

I REMEMBER, FROM my time at the Charité, one elderly patient who was slightly confused and had been wandering around the complex aimlessly until he finally ended up in Emergency. His blood values signaled a serious kidney problem, so I, being on duty, was contacted. The man seemed to me to be a bit disoriented but spoke in a friendly manner and didn't have any other complaints. "Just with peeing—that doesn't work as well as in earlier days," he admitted. Even without an ultrasound I could recognize a form the shape of a soccer ball where his kidneys were supposed to be. In the course of the sonography, I could see, as expected, a huge black hole full of roughly 6 pints—3 liters—of urine. Deep beneath it his prostate was no less impressive, with a volume of roughly 80 cc. Both kidneys were bloated and seriously blocked. Urine was no longer able to flow down the urethra to the chock-full bladder.

Kidney damage like this will have developed over the years without signs of pain or being in any other way apparent. Patients become symptomatic only as the kidneys' ability to detoxify becomes increasingly impaired. Rising urea levels in the blood over the years are often manifested by disorientation, as the urea—normally cleared by the kidneys into urine—can damage nerve cells. The unusual thing about this particular elderly gentleman was that he was wearing a white coat. He was a professor at the hospital.

This was, admittedly, an unusual case. Normally, we find that patients with such pronounced complications come to their urologist earlier.

When using ultrasound on the prostate, the structure of the tissue can be assessed only superficially. Calcifications or lesions are noticeable because they appear to be whitish under ultrasound. From a certain age on, almost every man has such deposits in the prostate. Because many of these patients are generally symptom-free and the lesions are found more by chance—for instance, during a medical checkup—it is rather unlikely that those lesions are directly linked to any problems. However, calcifications found clogging the excretory ducts of the prostate are thought to provoke inflammation in the prostate. Chronic causes of inflammation like this in turn increase the risk of malignant degeneration. These assumptions are probably justified, as they're based on data from huge studies. But ultimately, as part of the design of men, every man has a prostate and almost every man has, at some point in time, a greater or lesser degree of calcification in the gland. Anyway, as more than 50 percent of us men will eventually suffer from prostate cancer—don't panic, that number is put into context later in the chapter!—in my opinion it's futile to make a statistical connection between prostate calcification and prostate cancer.

The most important symptom when considering treatment options with the patient is his degree of distress. If he has to go to the bathroom during the night, if at a bar he spends thirty instead of twenty seconds at the urinal, if he can subdue the urge to pee for only twenty minutes instead of an hour—none of these are dramatic changes that are absolutely necessary to treat. Some people manage better than others. Questionnaires to measure the patient's degree of suffering can assist in estimating the effect of an individual's peeing performance on his quality of life. According to the textbooks and international guidelines, treatment should begin above a certain threshold. In practice, I've found it useful to ask the patients three simple additional questions about his symptoms:

1. Have you noticed any changes when you pee?
2. Are you worried about these changes?
3. Do you suffer from these changes?

Patients mostly notice the changes without any feelings of distress. They're often helped by an analogy to a different aspect of aging: over the years the temples become grayer or the hair sparser. These problems are also seldom treated. Bladder capacity changes with time, for almost everybody, but certainly doesn't always require treatment.

If two or three answers to these questions are "yes," then a variety of treatment options can be offered.

TREATMENT

The first symptom, having to go pee at night, is often stressful. Besides the prostate, the heart's diminishing pumping power, particularly in elderly men, can be another factor to take into consideration. If the heart is healthy, then some simple changes in daily routine can lead to an improvement in nighttime forays to the bathroom. All liquids that go in must come out again, but the last beer while watching the late-night talk shows doesn't immediately end up in the bladder. Drinks land first in the stomach. From there they flow into the gut for a time, where the beer is reabsorbed into the bloodstream. Our doughty heart muscles pump, day and night, roughly 10 to 15 pints (5 to 7 liters) of blood through the body and our kidneys. There the liquid is filtered off, little by little, until finally it ends up in the bladder as urine. Once the bladder is full enough, the urge to pass water increases—for people with higher bladder volumes, later, for others sooner. So it takes some time until the beer is ready for voiding. Depending on individual situations, a number of hours can pass between "in" and "out." When some patients claim that a drink they just consumed—in Cologne, that's normally a not-so-high-alcohol beer—goes directly into the drainage systems, they are only partially right. If the bladder is already full and liquids from the last round are added, then sometimes a reflex arc is initiated. Without taking the usual route from A to B—via the stomach, gut, bloodstream, and kidneys to the bladder—even the act of drinking a beer sends a message directly to the bladder: *Open the locks, there's more on the way!* Sometimes, as everyone knows, all you need to do is turn on a faucet to get the bladder in the mood.

Getting rid of the nighttime visit to the toilet means changing your drinking habits. Make sure the amount of liquids you get stays at around 4 pints (2 liters), but drink it earlier in the day. And stop drinking liquids after a certain time. Try stopping at 8 p.m., 7 p.m., or even earlier. Calculate the two to three hours it takes for the last liquids consumed to reach the bladder with your normal bedtime in mind. When, before going to sleep, you empty your bladder for the last time, based on your Stephen Hawking-level calculations there shouldn't be much more emptying to follow. Maybe this won't work out the first or second night—after all, we're not robots with a time switch. Nevertheless, with a bit of practice and discipline, a shift in your drinking habits should have a noticeable effect on the situation.

If you can't forgo your evening cup of tea while reading or if your peeing performance during the day has become worse, a number of herbal products can alleviate the situation. Mind you, scientific studies carried out on phytotherapeutic extracts (medically researched herbals) have shown that the active agents are far less effective than prescription drugs. Some studies show that the effects of herbal products are no different from those of placebos. My opinion on all this? First, you don't have to rigidly follow the findings of every study—results can sometimes be misleading. Second, the active ingredients of herbal remedies have considerably fewer side effects, so I can say with a clear conscience: just try them. Finally, I'm pretty thankful for the placebo effect. Patients are not being made fun of by placebos, as some people believe. A placebo effect can sometimes achieve a marked improvement. *Placebo* doesn't mean "I shall please" in the original Latin for nothing. And if it does please, why not continue to profit from it? You can take the active ingredients of extracts of the saw palmetto, stinging nettles, squashes, *Prunus africana* (the African cherry), and rye pollen, either individually or in combination. Squash seeds alone make little difference, unless used as a placebo.

The drugs I most often prescribe in my practice are related to the alpha-1 adrenergic receptor class of drugs— alpha blockers (α-blockers) for short. Here there are a number of candidates, with good old tamsulosin (Flomax) as my front-runner. The alpha blockers trigger relaxation of the muscles in the prostate, the bladder outlet, and the urethra, facilitating the voiding of the bladder. Because the alpha receptors are found not only in the bladder but also in the heart, blood pressure has to be monitored when using the drug. In some cases the blood pressure in the vascular system drops so dramatically that patients become dizzy, sometimes to the extent of blacking out. If patients are already taking antihypertensive drugs for high blood pressure, then these should, after consultation with the internist, be discontinued or prescribed in lower doses.

A further problem of treatment with alpha blockers is that there could be changes in ejaculation. Often the strength of ejaculation is considerably weakened, and a weary dribble certainly won't make an orgasm better. Sometimes on climaxing *nothing* comes out, as the prostate secretions disappear in the bladder (this is called *retrograde ejaculation*) or remain in the prostate (*anejaculation*). In both cases the orgasm doesn't feel right; ditto the pressure wave accompanying the semen shooting through the urethra. Here too it's worth trying treatment with alpha blockers. If the side effects described above appear, it's usually within forty-eight hours, and they disappear just as quickly after discontinuation of the drugs.

Tadalafil is a recent addition to the treatment options for prostate complaints. Besides improvements to bladder-voiding dysfunctions, other positive changes to andrological disorders are expected from tadalafil. The medication, however, is very expensive and other treatments are generally tried first.

A completely different approach for improving bladder capacity is to medicinally reduce the size of the prostate. The alpha blockers already described reduce the pressure on the prostate and urethra by relaxing the muscles in the discharging urinary tracts. The 5α-reductase inhibitors (finasteride and dutasteride) contract the organ by suppressing the testosterone metabolism in the prostate, which enables voiding of the bladder. Treatment can delay or prevent the necessity of surgery on an enlarged prostate, but the course of the treatment lasts up to eighteen months. Changes in testosterone balance can also lead to more or less unpleasant side effects. On the bright side, lowering testosterone metabolism can greatly reduce the chances of developing a malignant prostate tumor. If, however, a tumor does appear during treatment, then according to the research, it's going to be much more aggressive. Where there is light, there is shadow...

SURGICAL OPTIONS

In most cases the medical treatment options in the previous section are enough to solve bladder-emptying disorders. But if they all prove inadequate, there's a range of tried and true operative procedures to "slice up the pee drain," as my former boss was so fond of saying. The wealth of surgical possibilities would require a separate book. The gold standard of these intrusions is, without a doubt, transurethral resection of the prostate, commonly known as TURP, which involves removing tissue by electrocautery (also called *thermal cautery*) and inserting a catheter through the urethra to drain the bladder.

A number of technical innovations have led to a steady improvement in surgical methods. We also now have all kinds of laser operations in which the prostate is dissolved, shot at, or vaporized. Each method jostles for the best peeing results while attempting to have the lowest rate of complications.

Besides the pure surgical approaches is a range of endeavors to control the prostate using chemical or physical therapy. One recently developed procedure replaces the lateral lobes of the prostate, unblocking the urinary tract. My tip: whatever treatment you're being offered, first consider whether all the medicinal options have been exhausted. Postoperative complications, agreed, are rare, but once they arise, the aftereffects can often not be reversed, and if they *can* be reversed, then the process to do so is extremely complex.

Prostate Complaints of the Young

THE YOUNGEST PATIENTS who come to my practice and tell me about hitherto unknown peeing problems in the southern regions of their bodies are just learning to drive, doing their high school diploma, or finishing their apprenticeships. I can well remember the words of my urology lecturer at the University of Göttingen: "Prostate problems are afflictions not of old men but of aging men."

While working at various university hospitals, I hardly had any contact with young patients. The combination of the words "prostate" and "hospital" inevitably meant the operating theater, and 20-year-olds definitely don't need an operation. Only on moving to private practice, when the whole wide universe of urological diseases, symptoms, and sensitivities unfolded in front of me, did the words of that former professor come back to me from the murky depths of my mind. And how right he was.

Every week a number of patients under 30 come to my practice with LUTS, or lower urinary tract syndrome: problems passing water. The complaints are similar to those of men who could be their fathers—having to urinate frequently, dribbling, feeling a persistent urge to urinate, having a poor urine stream, passing urine during the night, and so on. The problem is that with this patient group, in all probability, nothing can be found by diagnostic investigation.

Generally, we carry out an ultrasound scan of these patients' bladder and prostate, run laboratory tests on their urine, and measure their urine stream pressure with a special toilet, all to exclude worst-case scenarios. In doing so, tumors, infections, and anatomical changes such as narrowing of the urethra can be mostly eliminated. Indeed, 99 percent of the time we find no pathological indications, which is a great relief to the patient.

Afterward I ask patients to keep a micturition diary for a few days. A micturition diary documents the time and the quantity of liquids consumed—the amounts drunk at a particular time—and the time and quantity of liquids leaving the bladder—the amounts of urine at a particular time. Unfortunately, keeping this diary means that the patient has to spend the next few days walking around with a measuring cup as faithful companion, ready to measure to the milliliter the amounts of urine at every visit to the washroom, which then have to be duly recorded. For the patient it's time-consuming and a bit annoying, but it's immensely helpful. We end up with a table covered with pages of precise information about inflow and outflow. These records can give the all-clear signal to three-quarters of the patients, meaning the data on liquid intake and toilet-visiting frequency and the bladder capacity that we can calculate from these findings lie in the safe middle range.

From patients' descriptions of their daily routine, it's noticeable that a third of them seem to be under considerable stress, and that this could be the real reason for frequent visits to the tiled room. Like the stomach, the bladder is an organ that registers stress and can rebel. And this doesn't only apply to the "stronger" sex—women can be afflicted too. For the rest of the patients, there can be no therapeutic solutions because there was literally nothing to be found. Sometimes the herbal remedies mentioned earlier can help, or we can make an appointment for a follow-up visit after the obligatory three months' wait. Often the problem is all over or forgotten by then.

CPPS: Chronic Pelvic Pain Syndrome

IF, IN ADDITION to problems with passing water, a patient has permanent pain in the region of the pelvis, this may be related to a separate condition: chronic pelvic pain syndrome, or CPPS for short. Before coming to this diagnosis, a prostate tumor or chronic bacterial inflammation should be ruled out. Frequent prostate inflammation can favor or trigger the syndrome, but bacteria aren't found in chronic cases. The pain is caused by chronic inflammatory changes to the muscle fascia or certain tendons that form, among other things, the thick plate of muscles on the pelvis to which the prostate is attached. If the pain remains chronic over months and years, the patient's quality of life is severely affected. Sometimes, in addition to pain in the lower abdomen, patients suffer from depression. I know of one case where a CPPS patient, out of desperation, tried to commit suicide.

Besides alpha blockers, anti-inflammatories, and herbal remedies, neurologically effective drugs can be used and have proven successful in countering the disease. Targeted nonmedicinal measures offer some relief, as the disease is a disruption of muscular and tendon structures of the pelvis. Physiotherapy, osteopathic treatment, biofeedback therapy, and extracorporeal shock wave therapy (ESWT) can lead to great improvements in the pelvic region.

Recently an outstandingly nice elderly gentleman came to our practice. We immediately got on well, and during the friendly banter almost forgot why he was actually here. He told me about his complaints in his groins, lower abdomen, scrotum, and penis. *Great*, I thought. *The whole broad spectrum of urology concentrated in one patient.* His description of the complaints was not really conducive to a proper diagnosis, so the next move was to check the exterior, and I started the search. I found one or another material weakness, but as men of 70 go, this gentleman would have no problem passing his urological test. In the ultrasound scan, however, I noticed an unusually full bladder. *Haven't I just seen the urine findings on the computer?* flashed through my mind, and I asked the man whether he had just given us a urine sample.

"Yes, yes," he answered. "But anyway, I have to go to the toilet every thirty minutes. Your receptionist handed me a beaker as soon as I arrived." With a waiting-room time of some fifteen minutes, it couldn't have been *that* long ago that the nice old man had had a pee. But then why was there so much urine in the bladder? And I had the first clue about the cause of his problem: the prostate, that rogue among organs!

We started with a course of tamsulosin, the usual starter drug of the alpha blockers. Two days later, I received a call. The drug was a great help, but the gentleman was so dizzy that he felt as if he were wandering around under remote control. So the prostate was indeed the culprit: all we had to do now was find a suitable treatment. Two other alpha blockers were no more help or even exacerbated the drop in blood pressure, so they could be eliminated as a treatment option. The prostate was far too small for 5α-reductase inhibitor therapy, so in this case they couldn't be considered. At the next appointment we went through the remaining options.

Surgery at this point was, in the opinion of the patient (and me), out of the question, so I decided on a new drug, which actually wasn't that new but had only just been approved for use for prostate disorders. At the beginning of a new therapy, I prescribe only short-term doses, so I can keep an eye on the side effects. After a month, if necessary, the patient can contact me and, assuming all is well, get a renewal for a further three months. To my surprise, after renewing the prescription, this gentleman asked for a new appointment and, to my even greater surprise, arrived together with his wife. Without uttering a word, she plonked a bottle of the finest Champagne on my desk while smiling at me serenely. "Well, I guess you're pretty happy with the choice of medication, then?" I said, looking forward to the contents of the bottle.

"You can't imagine how it has changed our lives," she said. "At last my husband can sleep almost throughout the night, and we can do things together without constantly having to be on the lookout for restrooms."

"And other things are happening again," added the nice old man, lovingly prodding his wife.

Happy down below—how apt!

Prostate Cancer

UP TO NOW we've concentrated on functional problems of the prostate that cause a deterioration in urination, but the prostate is also *the* male organ that most frequently degenerates and causes cancerous diseases. In Germany alone 60,000 new cases are diagnosed every year, about 160,000 in the United States. This figure climbs constantly because of improvements in diagnosis. The question is whether all such tumors should be found in the first place. There are studies in which the bodies of 80-year-olds and men even older were examined after a natural, non-cancer-related death. Although during their lives they had never been diagnosed with prostate cancer, prostate cancer was later identified in over 50 percent of cases. Who knows how long the gentlemen might have lived had they not suffered from heart attacks—despite prostate cancer?

On the other hand, there are over 10,000 deaths every year in Germany that are directly linked to prostate cancer, over 25,000 in the United States. So what do you do? Should you follow up on even the slightest suspicion just to be sure, and treat every diagnosed tumor with all the available means? I have my doubts. In order to get a comprehensive picture of the figures on, diagnostic options for, and treatment of prostate cancer, I recommend reading the National Comprehensive Cancer Network's prostate guidelines for patients, available at the NCCN website. If you type those terms into the search engine of your choice, you'll quickly find a PDF file of over a hundred pages, written in unbiased, understandable language, describing everything a layperson or patient could ever wish to know about the topic. With the diversity of treatment options even for malignant prostate cancer, unbiased descriptions are not altogether unimportant. Of course, sometimes individual situations are not covered by books or statistics, and then a confidential discussion with a urologist is necessary.

There are a number of general factors that you should know about when assessing prostate diseases. Prostate cancer, agreed, is a very common disease, but it often can be successfully treated. Even without therapy it isn't an inescapable death sentence. Often there aren't even symptoms. There are, however, a few malignant and many fewer *very* malignant forms of the cancer. It's important to distinguish which form we are dealing with. If a younger man has a suspected tumor, then it's likely to be malignant. As younger men can generally expect to have long remaining lifespans, it makes sense to gather information about precise diagnoses and longer-lasting forms of treatment. At the other end of the scale, it doesn't make much sense for an 85-year-old patient with a serious cardiac condition and without any symptoms who, by chance, has been diagnosed with a minor tumor to be given the full treatment. Of course, each case has to be seen and handled individually; nevertheless, there are age-related trends with the pathophysiology of prostate tumors.

SCREENING: WHEN AND HOW

As I've said, our ability to diagnose prostate cancer is constantly improving. Just recently a fusion between ultrasound and magnetic resonance imaging (MRI) has offered the possibility of discovering small tumors and removing them with targeted biopsies. Once this procedure becomes a part of the diagnostic routine, the incidence of new cases is likely to rise more dramatically than it already has. New approaches enable cases to be diagnosed that had been previously overlooked.

It's still unusual in the research to find someone under 45 being diagnosed with prostate cancer. I've had two patients below that age. Generally, I recommend screening for patients beginning at 40. This doesn't mean that from this point you have to be screened every year, but rather that you can establish a baseline early on, after which it is theoretically possible to spot the beginning of a tumor. If your risk factor at this point is nonexistent, as in most cases, then screening every five years is usually more than adequate. If, however, there are signs that you might have a higher risk factor, then screening every year or two is warranted. Depending on the findings over the years, fewer screenings can be carried out without waking any sleeping dogs.

What do reasonable precautions involve? Many people know that PSA levels are tumor markers. PSA stands for *prostate-specific antigens*, which are produced in the prostate regardless of whether it is healthy, diseased, enlarged, or old. Maybe you've already guessed that PSA levels can hinge on prostate size. As PSA values are not tumor specific but prostate specific, an enlarged prostate, for instance, will regularly provide higher readings. To put it another way, your PSA level alone is not really informative. Still, that measurement can be reinforced with a few others. Moreover, prostate tumors can be more conclusively diagnosed as one ages. Calculating the PSA ratio is another factor which makes the screening process considerably more valid. The PSA ratio reveals the amount of total PSA in the bloodstream in relation to protein-bound PSA. The smaller the ratio, the higher the risk of a tumor.

Let's sum up: Once we have the readings of the total PSA, the PSA ratio, the patient's age, and the size of the prostate, which can easily be measured with an ultrasound scan of the lower abdomen, the individual risk of prostate cancer can then be calculated. If, on the basis of the data, a specific risk is identified, a second screening should follow within a couple of weeks or months. If the risks remain the same or have even increased, then, in consultation with the patient, other measures can be considered.

We often end up at a point where a further diagnosis is necessary, to be sure about confirming or ruling out a tumor. Up until a few years ago, a biopsy—tissue sampling—of the prostate was the normal procedure for this. There are a number of ways of carrying out a prostate biopsy to get relevant information from the pathologist who examines the sample. Earlier, a biopsy would be performed on both sides of the prostate; nowadays the trend is the bigger the prostate, the more biopsies. A number of studies have pointed out that after forty-five or so core needle biopsies, at some stage very little prostate tissue remains. Tissue sampling is pretty much a hit-or-miss affair, and despite ultrasound scans, you can never be sure where a tumor is located in the prostate. The whole prostate gets punctured from back to front in the hope of hitting the tumor with one core or another. Which raises the question: If it takes forty biopsies to tease out the smallest of tumors, does that tumor really have to be treated or even discovered? Patients should also be fully informed about the risk of severe inflammation, as biopsies are usually carried out with the aid of transanal ultrasound and a long core needle is inserted through the wall of the rectum and into the prostate to get samples. Of course, all needless biopsies should be avoided if possible in view of these possible complications, which can end in long stays in intensive care or even worse.

For a long time, researchers have tried to include improved imaging techniques in the diagnosis of prostate tumors in order to carry out pinpoint biopsies. The usual ultrasounds of the abdomen or via a rectal probe are not enough to localize a tumor in the prostate with absolute certainty. Computer programs that process ultrasound images are meant to facilitate the discovery of areas of the prostate with suspected tumors. Some procedures have produced good data, others not so good. Nothing yet could be termed a long-lasting or resounding success. A couple of years ago, radiologists began carrying out tests using magnetic resonance imaging. MRI is well suited for assessing soft tissue structures. What's more, tumor tissues have different signaling characteristics from healthy tissue, and metabolism in tumors is also different and can be recognized by MRI. There are now very good MRI procedures that assess risk using prostate imaging reporting and data system (PIRADS) classification. But even the highest risk bracket, PIRAD 5, considers the presence of a tumor only "highly likely" and not "certain." Here too a biopsy is needed for a conclusive diagnosis.

In addition to the usual PSA levels, there are other markers that can indicate the presence of a prostate tumor. The PCA3 test, measuring the expression of prostate cancer gene 3 in urine samples, and the p2PSA test, which like the usual PSA test is carried out by a blood test, have both led to a slight improvement in the detection rate of tumors according to a number of studies, but for various reasons they have ultimately never become part of the daily clinical routine.

ACTIVE SURVEILLANCE

Should prostate cancer be discovered through screening, there is, as a rule, still no call for (over)hasty measures. Slow tumor growth rates normally allow the patient enough time to become informed about the wide range of treatment options and then to decide on the most suitable action. Here too I would recommend taking a thorough look at the NCCN guidelines for patients. They include a comprehensive overview of the possible treatments. In consultation with your urologist, you'll then be able to weigh the options and ultimately choose the right one for you. Your urologist shouldn't have a problem with your seeking a second opinion from another urologist and may well even encourage you to do so.

Until a few years ago, for patients up to a certain age, almost every prostate tumor was treated by some means or another. If after the pathologist's final postoperative tests on the organ few malignant cancer cells were found, the patient was considered lucky, as the chances of the disease progressing after treatment were considered very slim. But we have moved on. It has long been known that not all prostate tumors are troublesome, so we now try to single out the patients whose tumors aren't and spare them the treatment.

Patients with slightly less malignant cancer types who in their lives haven't experienced problems are offered active surveillance instead of treatment. This is quite a shift—up until a few years ago almost every patient was either operated on or irradiated. Active surveillance means that the patient is monitored every three months to appraise the development of the tumor. If the tumor remains stable, there's no need yet for treatment. Should there be changes in the tumor, and thus in the risks to the patient, things can still be calmly considered and the most suitable form of treatment chosen.

The treatment options for a newly discovered tumor—and here I mean in the first place tumors confined to the prostate, not ones that have spread—are surgery, radiation therapy, and other interventions.

SURGERY AND OTHER TREATMENT OPTIONS

During surgery for prostate cancer, the prostate and the attached seminal vesicles are removed. The urethra and bladder are then sewn back together so that the bladder can be voided as usual. Years ago, a prostatectomy involved a large cut in the pelvic zone (retropubic) or between your legs (perineal). About twenty years ago the age of laparoscopy began. This was just when I was completing my training in Berlin at the Charité, which had a worldwide reputation as a center of laparoscopic radical prostatectomy.

Later, robotic-assisted techniques developed from laparoscopy. Robotic-assisted procedures were originally conceived for the U.S. Army, to perform remote-controlled operations on injured soldiers in war zones. At the beginning of the 2000s, the civilian applications of these operations were recognized. Even though the operation really *is* performed by a robot, there's no reason to panic! The robot makes no independent movements and can't be programmed for just any old procedure. The operation is conducted by a urologist, who guides tiny robotic arms from a console into the patient's abdomen. The console, if necessary, can be many thousands of miles away, as long as the internet access has been paid for. The operator sees a 3-D image, many times enlarged, which is transmitted to the console's 3-D screen from a camera inside the patient's body. While the robot-assisted operation takes place deep below the pelvis, the surgeon sits, relaxed, at the ergonomically optimized high-tech machine and is able to perform surgical intrusions with the greatest precision.

In the early days, these operations took hours, and the learning curve at the beginning was not particularly steep. Today there are some fifty surgical robots in Germany alone, and the results of the operations are—and I can say this from my own experience—excellent. I have a number of patients who have had surgery using the da Vinci system. The high costs are certainly a problem that we will increasingly encounter in the future with the development of high-tech medical procedures. In general, though, I have to say that the results of operations performed by experienced surgeons using conventional manual methods don't have to be worse than robotic surgery. On the contrary, rather an open operation from an old hand than a robotic one from a greenhorn! But here too progress cannot be stopped, and at some stage every operator has to perform his first operation.

The risks of surgical removal of the prostate have been steadily decreasing in recent years. But there is still a risk after the surgery of suffering erectile dysfunction or incontinence.

Besides the surgical option, prostate tumors can also be successfully treated by radiation. The advantages are simple—you're spared the risks of surgical intervention. On the other hand, a tumor can recover after radiation and continue to grow. Depending on the stage and malignancy of the tumor, the right procedure has to be chosen to reduce the risks. At the moment there are two different forms of radiation therapy. *Percutaneous radiation* is carried out externally, through the skin. Then there is *brachytherapy*, in which radioactive "seeds" are placed directly inside the prostate. There are two distinct forms of brachytherapy: high dose and low dose. The most suitable option should be decided after consultation with a urologist. Problems can also crop up with radiation therapy, but here too rapid advances in medical technology in recent years have steadily reduced the rate of posttreatment complications. But still there can be gut and bladder problems and/or erectile dysfunction.

Just for the sake of completeness, I should mention the other interventions: hyperthermia, cryotherapy, and high-intensity focused ultrasound (HIFU). Here, attempts are made to treat prostate tumors using physical forces: heat, cold, and ultrasound. There have been signs of influences on the tumor, and probably there have been success stories with one option or another. None of these three treatment options, however, has been clinically proven to provide a lasting healing success, which is why they should be considered only in carefully selected individual cases or as part of a high-grade clinical trial with precise patient monitoring.

Cancer cells in the prostate don't react only to radiation. As most such tumors are dependent on the male sexual hormone testosterone, lowering testosterone levels can slow down tumor growth. The risks of radiation therapy or surgery are then dispensed with. Hormonal withdrawal sometimes has unpleasant side effects. Sometimes, however, it makes sense with advanced cases of tumors to use hormone therapy in conjunction with radiation treatment or after surgery.

However you look at it, prostate cancer is not a disease you would choose. Nevertheless, there is no reason for panic or despair when it's diagnosed. Nowadays, with the multitude of different treatment options, the chances of recovery are good and quality of life after therapy is mostly great.

three

WOMEN'S UROLOGY: DON'T WORRY, PEE HAPPY

IT MAY SEEM hard to believe, but at our all-male practice, one in every four patients is in fact female. Have the ladies landed here by mistake? No way! Ninety percent of these women suffer from the same affliction: bladder infections. Most women with bladder infections I don't even get to see—they've already been treated by their regular doctors or gynecologists. The big step to a urologist is only ventured if, after the fifth course of antibiotics, they notice that something is still not quite right.

Bladder infections are as varied as the Queen's clothes, the only constant being that they are damned painful. While this diagnosis is rather the exception for men—with similar symptoms, men are more likely to have an inflamed prostate—there are serious estimates that, at some stage in life, every other woman suffers from a bladder infection. This is the equivalent, give or take a bit, of a quarter of the world's population, and is easily high enough for one of the top spots in the top 10 most unpopular diagnoses. Normally, bacteria are the cause of these bladder infections, rarely fungi, parasites, or viruses.

Bladder Infections: Causes and Treatment

E. COLI

The most common pathogen is *Escherichia coli*, lovingly termed *E. coli* by the fraternity. Theodor Escherich discovered the bacterium in the late nineteenth century and described its role in the development of the immune system of infants.

Since then the image of *E. coli* as a benign bacterium has been severely dented. The little beast now enjoys the limelight solely as the cause of annoying, and often difficult to treat, infections. But *E. coli* is actually at home in the intestines and usually does a lot of good there, from stimulating immunity to preventing diarrhea to producing vitamins. Besides also triggering chronic gut infections, pathogens—the disease-causing strains of the bacterium—induce inflammations of the bladder mucous membrane, especially in women. The reason for the differences between the sexes in who gets bladder infections is anatomical: the differing length of the male and female urethra. Mr. Smith's can be 8 inches long (20 centimeters), whereas Mrs. Jones's might be just 1½ inches (4 centimeters). The bacteria have a considerably shorter journey in women, and they don't need to be asked twice. Furthermore, the gut and the urethra have sought out practically the same anatomical niche to exit the body. Once again, not really one of God's better ideas. He worked just as sloppily on the prostate, so as far as suffering goes, there is equality of the sexes.

This is also the reason that bladder infections often show up after sexual intercourse. It is sometimes assumed that men are the carriers of the pathogens and pass them on to women. In fact, however, the pathogens loiter in the vulval vestibule waiting for activities that will enable them to hitch a ride toward the urethra—and, incidentally, regardless of painstaking hygienic precautions. From the urethra, they go on to the bladder, nest in the mucous membrane, and do what they are good at doing: inflame. The typical symptoms are pain while peeing, pain after peeing, and sometimes pain between pees. In addition, frequent peeing, small amounts of pee, and sometimes blood in the pee. It has a lot to do with peeing, and it's very annoying. It becomes more than an inconvenience when partners separate because their sex life has ground to a halt, or when jobs are lost because half of the day had to be spent in the ladies' room.

DIAGNOSTICS

Symptoms alone are often enough to diagnose a bladder infection. Nevertheless, it is sometimes sensible to carry out further tests. Either you can be certain of the diagnosis or you can learn things that can be particularly helpful to urologists in choosing treatment. Some "expert" patients have home test kits to make their own diagnosis. These can be helpful, but you shouldn't put too much faith in urine dipsticks or test strips, as the results shown can be misleading: sometimes the patient feels as if she's suffering from a severe infection but the test results are crystal-clear negative, and other times they're plum purple but she's perfectly healthy. Both combinations are possible, but the results don't exactly help the patient to understand her illness.

In our practice, on top of a dipstick urine test, we always run a microscopic analysis. In this process, the urine is placed in a centrifuge, and then the clumps of cells that settle at the bottom of the centrifuge tubes are smeared onto a specimen slide and analyzed in the lab at 400× magnification. Bacteria, infected cells and blood cells, mucosa cells, fungi, and specific parasites in the urine can be identified. The findings are considerably more meaningful and reliable than the test sticks could ever be.

On top of this, for every urine sample we see a pathogen in, we start up a bacteria culture, to multiply the pathogen for identification. When we've discovered the first and last names of the beast, we do a resistogram typing. Here the resistance and sensitivity of the troublemaker is tested against eight of the most common antibiotics. If the bacteria are resistant to one of the typical antibiotics, there's no point in prescribing it. If after two treatment cycles with a particular antibiotic the patient is still suffering from complaints—there you go, you may be dealing with antibiotic resistance. I can well remember the patient totally desperate and with tears in her eyes who emptied onto my desk a Walmart bag full of empty pill bottles from antibiotics she'd been prescribed by a variety of sources over the year, without anyone having thought to name the bacterium or test its resistance.

THERAPY: WATER AND PLANTS

So what to do when you have a burning sensation when you pee and the restroom doesn't get any prettier after the twentieth visit? You don't have to immediately go for the antibiotics. On the contrary: it makes a lot of sense to first treat the infection by drinking more liquids. Several studies have shown that simple bladder infections can be effectively treated with an increased intake of liquids. They don't have to be those nasty-tasting bladder and kidney teas—water is fine. The occasional beer or wine spritzer would also do the trick as long as the immune system doesn't nose-dive.

If water intake proves insufficient, it still doesn't mean you have to resort to the pharmaceutical arsenal. Plenty of plant-based agents have proven, individually or in combination, to have good effects on bladder infections. One of the best-known herbs to use against acute bladder infections is the common bearberry (*Arctostaphylos uva-ursi*), the leaves of which are offered in a variety of forms—lozenges, pills, and juice. Alternatively, goldenrod (*Solidago virgaurea*), besides having an anti-inflammatory effect, also flushes the urethra and can be used for long-term treatment or as a precautionary measure. A good combination is nasturtium (*Tropaeolum majus*) and horseradish root; high doses have produced good results in the treatment of acute bladder infections. Conveniently, this old household remedy from the herb garden has also proven useful even in low dosages: after repeated infections, the combination can be useful as a preventive after sexual intercourse. Extract of field horsetail (*Equisetum arvense*) also has anti-inflammatory effects and can be combined with extract of fumitory (*Fumaria officinalis*), an anticonvulsant.

Cranberries are widely used as a therapy for bladder infections but unfortunately mostly used wrongly. The proanthocyanidin in the berries has an antibiotic effect similar to chocolate or a plate of French fries—namely, none whatsoever. Cranberry juice or its dried extract do not act against the bacteria but form a protective layer on the bladder's mucous membrane, which prevents *E. coli* from adhering and thus causing inflammatory reactions. Once symptoms are present, cranberry therapy makes little sense, as the bacteria have reached their objective and are already established on the bladder wall. The sour berries, however, are an effective prophylaxis—a preventive measure—when used at the right time. This means regularly and over the long term. Like most plant-based products, cranberry juice is not covered by health insurance, so regular use over two to three months means that costs mount.

ANTIBIOTICS

Once a bladder infection is present, and if drinking more liquid and taking herbal substances is insufficient to shake it off, then antibiotic treatment is, of course, a good and worthwhile means of effecting a speedy recovery. There are plenty of antibiotics on the market, but you have to choose just one, preferably the right one. Guidelines published by the German and European urology associations suggest which antibiotics are suitable for specific situations, but it seems to me that most doctors don't follow them. Yet it's not complicated. As long as there's no antibiogram indicating resistance or signs of other complications, the solution is simple, because you have to look for only two active ingredients: fosfomycin and nitrofurantoin. Should there be signs of allergic reactions or these drugs have proved ineffective during previous treatment phases, then, of course, other antibiotics can be taken, but the bacterium causing the infection and whether it is treatment-resistant must be determined first.

The Worst-Case Scenario: Chronic Recurrent Bladder Infection

UNFORTUNATELY *E. COLI* BACTERIA have acquired a bad habit that makes treatment with antibiotics considerably more difficult. The bacteria, after having caused a respectable infection, bond together in mucosal cell vesicles and form colonies. These bubble-like structures, filled with bacteria, separate from the surface of the bladder mucous membrane and dive deep into the center of the cell. In the depths of this dark pond they are well protected from antibiotics. Once the treatment has been completed, the little bubbles, together with the bacteria, return to the surface, the outer layer of the bubbles merges with the bladder mucosa, and the infection starts all over again. There's no new bladder infection as such—it's just the old bacteria creeping out of their hideout and causing further havoc.

The therapeutic approach against this bacterial strategy has been known for a number of years but is very seldom applied. Forskolin, the extract of the plant Indian coleus (*Plectranthus barbatus*), ensures that the bacteria-filled bubbles are brought to the surface of the mucous membrane. The outer layer of the bacteria's home bonds again with the surface of the bladder wall, and the bacteria are flushed out into the interior of the bladder. This way the bacteria are exposed to the antibiotics, and treatment becomes effective. Forskolin can't be bought in drug stores. You can get it either at health food stores or online. Forskolin also has a small side effect, positive for most people: it's active in fat metabolism, meaning that it may help exercise lead to weight loss.

There is another method for killing off a recurrent bladder infection. D-mannose is a special form of sugar that is ignored by metabolism and directly excreted in the urine. D-mannose is available in capsule and powder form (which can be mixed with juice) and is taken several times a day. In the bladder D-mannose binds to *E. coli*, preventing it from clamping to the bladder wall. With sufficient liquid intake the free-swimming beasties are, bit by bit, peed out of the bladder. Scientific studies are currently being conducted on both forskolin and D-mannose, but reliable results will be known only in a few years.

To sum up, patients suffering from recurrent bladder infections have the following recommendations: mornings and evenings, 125 milligrams of forskolin; 2,000 milligrams of d-mannose a day; goldenrod extract for flushing purposes with at least eight 8-ounce glasses (2 liters) of liquid a day. Healing the bladder can cost quite a bit and the routine should be maintained for a few weeks, but at least, in my experience, there's a high response rate.

Preventing Bladder Infections

HYGIENE

The best thing is not to have a bladder infection in the first place. But no matter what preventive measures you take, bladder infections will not vanish from your life overnight. Sometimes it takes weeks or months to detect a trend. But the more you take care of yourself and take preventive measures, the less often you'll suffer from bladder infections.

So what can you do to avoid an infection? Excessive hygiene measures aren't particularly appropriate for the time being, but take care to avoid chemical substances for intimate hygiene. Often pH levels in the mucous membrane of the vagina are damaged by intimate lotions, and heavily perfumed shower gels disrupt the body's own defenses. Most of the time, regular washing with warm water is perfectly adequate. As mentioned earlier, the typical agents of bladder infections live in the gut. In the dear God's anatomic blueprint for women, the bowels and the urethra are neighbors, and sometimes neighborly relations are strained. It should be taken for granted that after a visit to the restroom, the right direction for wiping is *not* toward the urethra, at the front.

You should also consider whether your underwear really has to be made of synthetic materials or silk, both of which create a warm, moist climate in the genital region and, more importantly, can be washed only at lower temperatures. Cotton is a breathable fabric and the residual germs on it can be washed out at considerably higher temperatures. A small amount of vinegar in the washing machine does the rest.

SEXUAL HYGIENE

Bladder infections often appear after sex. I've had despairing women in my practice because normal relations were simply no longer possible.

Condoms don't help prevent bladder infections—bacteria are still transported from the vaginal vestibule to the urethra. Still, if a condom slips and a man's partner develops an infection, the man should go for a checkup. Maybe he has an infection of the seminal tract that's been passed on to his partner. Urethral swabs and urine and semen samples will quickly provide the answers.

That said, the transmission of infection from man to woman is pretty unusual. Should you have no (medical) complaints after having had intercourse using condoms with a man who has been tested for infection and been cleared, then your problem might be an allergic reaction. In very rare cases, the diagnosis is seminal hypersensitivity—an allergic reaction to some constituent of the semen. To determine this, the person having the reaction can take an antihistamine or use a vaginal anti-allergen spray before intercourse. Discomfort after sex should improve without having to slip on rubber protection.

There are also a number of different measures to avoid increasing the amount of bacteria in the urethra. Although it sounds a bit dirtier than it is, one simple but highly effective method is sex with a full bladder. The pelvic floor and the inner bladder sphincter muscle, for obvious reasons, have to really make an effort to restrain the urethra, which automatically impedes bacteria from entering the bladder. For those of you who find this method unappetizing, a 1990s study showed that a full bladder increases sexual arousal.

The other method of automatically closing the urethra is probably a little more pleasant. The female urethra, like the male one, is enclosed in erectile tissue, and this tissue also expands as sexual urge increases. During a lecture by a female specialist in sexual medicine, I learned that the occurrence of bladder infections was diametrically opposed to the amount of foreplay! So give yourself plenty of time. Unfortunately, I couldn't find the corresponding study during my research. If, however, she's right about the correlation, then the idea could be taken further. Phosphodiesterase 5 inhibitors (PDE5), which have been proven to improve circulation in the male cavernous body, could be used by women to avoid after-sex infections by restricting the urethra—Viagra as prevention of infection.

ANTIBIOTICS AS PREVENTIVE

Even if it's not mentioned in the textbooks and, from a microbiological standpoint, is not actually permitted, one-off prophylactic antibiotic therapy can make sense in certain cases. Studies on women suffering from recurrent bladder infections who take a single antibiotic dose just before intercourse have shown good results. In our student days we learned that such procedures, in the medium and long term, caused antibiotic resistance and, in the end, more problems than at the beginning. When, however, there are *no* other options, when there's no history of antibiotic intolerance, and when the treatment actually helps, then from a medical point of view, nothing can be said against it. Two smaller studies of pre-sex antibiotic use have shown a sixfold reduction in after-sex bladder infection. *If* smaller studies can be trusted ...

Another option for reducing infections—again not to be found in textbooks—is regular administration of an antibiotic every ten to fourteen days regardless of sexual activity. Here too there has been little scientific research, so the risks of long-term treatment haven't been tested.

One antibiotic therapeutic method, however, *has* made it into the textbooks. A number of my patients have profited from three months of treatment with low doses of nitrofurantoin, sold under the trade name Macrobid. If the troublemakers causing the infection have been identified and are sensitive to nitrofurantoin, then after three to five days, twelve weeks of a small maintenance dose can be started, taken before going to bed. Sometimes a significant reduction in the number of bladder infections can be seen from following this regimen. If this is accompanied by the plant-based therapy options mentioned above, then, ideally, the effects of both will add together.

IMMUNIZATION

Often in female patients suffering from recurrent bladder infections an immune-response factor is suspected. Some consideration to this line of inquiry is not totally unwarranted—after all, a significantly higher proportion of women never or very seldom suffer from recurrent bladder infections. The spectrum of the typical pathogens is, luckily, relatively small, so focusing on the usual bowel suspects and a couple of other likely candidates seems sensible for a general improvement in the immune status.

Here the market has a number of options for bolstering the immune system against *E. coli* and company. One popular method consists of a course of tablets that lasts nine months—for this very reason not one of my favored immunotherapies. The regularity and length of treatment present many patients with practically unsolvable problems. These begin with the very human tendency, from time to time, to forget unpleasant things (limiting the success of immunization) and end at the latest when taking a pill clashes with the desire for a garden barbecue, a banana split, or a bag of chips. In other words, there are better treatment models.

There are, for example, intramuscular injections, as in childhood vaccinations. Over three to six weeks the patient has three injections, to the upper arm or the bottom, containing a vaccine against *E. coli* and its friends. Occasionally there are side effects—cold symptoms, pains at the puncture site, and sometimes even bladder infection symptoms. The outcome, however, is more lasting, in my opinion, and full implementation of the vaccine is far more likely than with the tablet option.

Should the industrially produced vaccines have no effect whatsoever, you could try specific immunotherapy. In this, a stool sample of the patient is used to make a personalized vaccine that corresponds to the patient's bacterial spectrum.

Here too, as with all preventive measures, there are no guarantees that you will never again be troubled by bladder infections. A clear reduction in their frequency or a lessening of symptoms would also be worth considering a partial success. Especially with immunotherapy, some time has to pass before you can be sure of the treatment's effectiveness: allow a year before passing final judgment.

GENERAL IMMUNITY

I don't subscribe readily to the adage "A healthy body is never ill," but it's advisable to live "healthily" in order to avoid regular infections. Your general immunity status is certainly a decisive factor on top of others when it comes to chronic bladder infections. Smoking, excessive alcohol consumption, and stress damage the immune system in the long run. Of course a healthy lifestyle, with physical activity, a balanced diet, not too much meat, and enough liquids, is the prerequisite for a healthy immune system. Maybe you're one of the lucky people without health problems, but still, if you want to do something for your immune system, I would like to briefly introduce a number of naturopathic and orthomolecular (supplement-based) options.

Vitamins are indispensable for a functioning immune system. Whether, as Nobel Prize winner and founder of orthomolecular therapy Linus Pauling suggested, it has to be 180 milligrams of vitamin C a day is questionable, but it has been scientifically proven that vitamin C supports the immune system and that 3,000 milligrams a day acidifies urine and thus has an antibacterial effect. Vitamin D is also an important factor in immunological health. The problem with vitamin D, however, is that sufficient amounts cannot be ingested from food alone—you would have to eat quite a lot of sardine sandwiches every day, as vitamin D is most commonly found in fish fats. The production of vitamin D in the skin depends on sun exposure. In northern and southern latitudes, far from the equator, it is not surprising to see figures that in many places 80 percent of men and 90 percent of women are vitamin D deficient. Several studies have linked vitamin D deficiency to an increased risk of bladder infections and recommended vitamin D supplements, at least in the darker winter months. In our clinic, we measure our patients' vitamin D levels and, depending on the degree of deficiency, recommend 1,000 to 2,000 units a day or 20,000 units once a week.

There are other possibilities of cranking up the immune system, using antioxidants. Antioxidants counteract the effects of free radicals. We're not talking here about anarchists but about parts of molecules created in complex reactions in all metabolic processes. Free radicals are, among other things, responsible for the development of cancer, aging processes, disruption to cellular metabolism, and weakening the immune system. Antioxidants can be found in more or less "healthy" foods such as coffee, beer, chocolate, and wine. High-dose therapy using these "therapeutic" agents, should, however, be avoided in the long run. But there are a number of blockbuster naturopathic and orthomolecular radical-scavengers that, in an appropriate therapy, can improve the immune system.

In addition to vitamins C and D, selenium is one of the most potent antioxidant radical-scavengers. Selenium is a trace element present in every human cell as well as in inanimate matter all over the world, and it has an important role in immune defense. Studies have shown that intensive care patients with severe septicemia had a lower mortality rate when treated with selenium. A selenium deficiency in otherwise healthy people has been shown to increase susceptibility to infections. In Germany, where I live, we have a problem. The soil on German farmlands has relatively low levels of selenium, so we often have to reckon with selenium deficiencies on top of the already mentioned vitamin D deficiencies. Scandinavian countries have similar problems with soil and have added selenium to manure. After a few years, the selenium levels in plants, animals, and therefore foodstuffs increase, and statistically higher levels of selenium have been measured in Norwegians' blood. Furthermore, the incidence of thyroid diseases decreased.

For people who wish to incorporate radical-scavengers in their diet, try this: one of the antioxidative heavyweights is contained in turmeric, a member of the South Asian ginger family. Anyone who's eaten a curry knows the yellowy-orange spice and its distinctive taste. The antioxidative effects of Ayurvedic cuisine multiply when cayenne is added. Many other antioxidants can also be incorporated into everyday cooking: red berries, ginger, and green tea are just a few of the biological secret weapons.

In traditional Chinese medicine (TCM) the intestines are often considered the hub of the immune system. Naturally, the intestines also play a leading role in bladder infections, as they are home to the typically involved bacteria. Many TCM specialists and naturopaths focus on intestine therapy in the treatment of symptoms of immunity deficiencies. There are umpteen natural options for keeping the intestines healthy. Basic eating habits have a positive effect on the intestines' immunological functions. Eat fewer meat and white flour products and more fruit and vegetables. A couple of spoonfuls of pure bran in your breakfast cereal is an excellent source of fiber. With this alone, your intestines will be happy after some weeks. If you want, you can support the intestines with probiotics such as lactobacillus, found in certain milk products. And one thing you should definitely do to enhance the intestines is to try to avoid antibiotics.

Pain without an Infection

HERE'S A SITUATION that often arises in my practice. A patient comes as an emergency case complaining about her bladder infection despite having taken various antibiotics. Examination, however, turns up no signs of infection from the urine test strip's chemical analysis and not even the slightest hint of pathological findings under the microscope. But the patient describes typical bladder infection symptoms. What to do now? Send her home with a clean bill of health? Refer her to a psychiatrist? Give her a course of yet another antibiotic?

I have to assume that the patient didn't have an overwhelming desire to visit a urologist and probably could do without the pain. I can safely conclude that her condition is as she describes it. When everything speaks against an acute infection but the symptoms suggest one, the answer often lies in the bladder wall's mucosal barrier. It's often difficult to judge whether this disruption has been caused by all the antibiotic treatments, by the infection itself, or by some other factor.

I think of the bladder's mucous membrane in these cases as weakened, breached, or raw. Whether it's because of bacteria or not, the bladder *hurts*, typically after passing water, when the wall of the emptied bladder deflates and the mucous membranes rub against each other. Long-term treatment options include the already mentioned cranberry extracts, to slowly strengthen the protective layer on the interior bladder wall. But if the pain is acute, two to three months of treatment is not really an option. Bladder instillation therapy is an effective and, above all, quick alternative measure. In instillation therapy a tube is inserted into the bladder and medication is infused through it to coat the bladder wall. The active ingredients of products for this on the market include components of the interior protective layers of the bladder. Glycosaminoglycan (GAG) layers cover the injured mucous membrane like a bandage, protecting it against irritation. Symptoms often improve after only one session. But to build up enough protection, the active ingredients should be infused at least four times in a month. Instillation therapy is a good way of achieving rapid recovery in complicated and severe cases. Unfortunately, not all health insurance systems cover it, and the treatment is not exactly inexpensive.

Reading between the lines in consultations with afflicted patients, I've found that bladder infections happen more often in times of stress. You've probably noticed a link between stress and problems peeing. The bladder sometimes acts like the psyche's plaything. If the link is patently obvious and the patient has an open ear to her psyche, then mental health treatment might make sense to discover the root causes. One method for confronting stress and its consequences is mindfulness-based stress reduction (MBSR). A sample program consists of eight weeks of two-hour workshops focusing on mindful awareness for stress management. From my own experience, I can say that a workshop like this can be very helpful and even fun.

four

INFERTILITY

MY CAREER IN andrology began during a coffee break in 2001 when a colleague at the Charité in Berlin asked me if I would take over his consultations with parents trying to have children. Albrecht had been offered a post as senior physician elsewhere and was about to leave the hospital. At that time I knew as much about this field as a cow knows about skateboarding, but I agreed, as there were some good nurses working in that clinic and I thought the daily routine would be more relaxed than on the wards. Albrecht also told me, almost incidentally, that people trying to become pregnant were basically very nice, grateful patients who deserved all the support they could get. And it's pretty much been like that. So, no sooner said than done. I gleaned some information from a couple of books over the weekend, and on the next Thursday morning I was suddenly the expert "baby enabler" in Europe's largest hospital.

After a few uncomplicated months, I had pretty much got the hang of things and was really enjoying the new task. The patients were young, healthy, and fit—unlike those of my colleagues, holding their weekly prostate cancer or incontinence sessions. I also noticed that the practicing urologists in Berlin were relieved that someone had taken on this field, a time-consuming area few of them really knew much about. Over the years I gathered a fair amount of expertise (for fun, my colleagues gave me the nickname The Sperminator—even doctors can scrape the barrel!) and positive feedback began to grow, including in the media. After the success of my 6 a.m. breakfast TV show *The Stork from Mitte* (Mitte is the central borough in Berlin), in which I would chat about and around the subject of infertility and its treatment, my consultancy sessions were bursting at the seams and extra sessions had to be organized. The subject has accompanied me now for fifteen years, and with some 10,000 semen analyses behind me I have managed to accumulate a fairly rich pool of experience.

Diagnosing Infertility

SO WHEN DO we call absence of pregnancy *infertility*? Statistically, 90 percent of couples wanting to get pregnant have their wish fulfilled within twelve months, and 95 percent are happy to announce incoming offspring after twenty-four. Infertility, by definition, is only an issue if pregnancy doesn't occur within a year with regular intercourse, with "regular" being defined in the literature as twice to three times a week.

The causes of infertility are equally found in men and women. Typically, however, it is almost always women who, in the absence of pregnancy, try to get to the bottom of the supposed infertility and visit their gynecologists. Regard-less of whether she receives dependable information from her visit, a trip to an andrologist should also be obligatory: without a spermiogram, the woman's diagnosis is only half the story. Should male problems be contributing to the fail-ure to conceive, then treatment for the woman, with its possible side effects, should proceed only after the man's reproductive capabilities have been reestablished.

There is a wide range of possible reasons for failures in paternity. Congenital or anatomic roots could be the rea-son for a change for the worse shown in spermiograms. For instance, during childhood one or both testicles might have failed to slip down the inguinal canal to the scrotum, and they have to be helped surgically. This ailment is called *bilateral funiculitis*, and leads to orchiopexy: more or less a groin hernia operation, as surgically the entry points are the same and "groin hernia" is far less of a mouthful.

Varicoceles are another classic anatomical cause. Up to 30 percent of men have a more or less abnormal enlarge-ment of the network of testicular blood vessels (the pampiniform venous plexus) in the scrotum. Sometimes you can feel varicoceles as a soft squidgy mass above the testicles, usually to the left, on account of the vascular anat-omy. If not, then ultrasound usually provides an answer; sometimes a Doppler test is also necessary. If you know what you're looking for, you can often identify a varico-cele both to the left of the testicles and to the right. This situation, however, has yet to gain an entry in the text-books where varicocele is still described as a unilateral (one-sided) disease.

Besides bilateral funiculitis and varicoceles, a range of possible genetic, infectious, medicinal, and hormonal causes have to be tested for. Environmental influences such as stress, heat, smoking, and an unhealthy lifestyle can also bring spermatogenesis—the creation of sperm—to a standstill. Often no clear cause can be found for bad spermiogram results, in which case we call it *idiopathic infertility*, *idiopathic* in doctor talk meaning "I haven't got a clue." If you consider how much professional and social stress has increased in the last decades, that there are estrogenizing softening agents in all plastic packaging, and that drinking water, thanks to the millions of prescriptions of the pill, contains considerably more female hormones than it used to, environmental influences on male fertility are hardly surprising.

But now I have to emphasize that a "bad" spermiogram is by no means a sign that the man will never have any offspring. Let's take a look at the current normal values of spermiograms. Your basic spermiogram consists of three important parameters: sperm quantity or, as the case may be, sperm density; motility, or the ability of the individual sperm cells to move; and finally morphology, the appearance of the sperm. (A few other aspects can be diagnostically useful, but more on those later.)

For each of the three elements, there are norms that were decided upon in a large international study. Researchers analyzed the spermiograms of thousands of men who, within a year and with no previous infertility diagnosis or therapeutic aids, had successfully initiated a pregnancy. Imagine a huge lake of sperm given a good stir and shaken a bit in order to calculate the scale for "normal" male fertility.

For patients whose spermiogram ratings are below the range of reference, the statistical chances of pregnancy are reduced. This doesn't mean, exactly, that they're absolutely incapable of reproducing. If, however, the ratings are progressively worse and worse over multiple spermiograms, then the chances of pregnancy are statistically so minimal that we have to assume infertility on the part of the man. As long as the microscope shows moving sperm, in principle, there is some chance of pregnancy, but just how great the chances are depends. Sometimes you need a little more investigation to move from the supposed to the real cause of infertility.

A Middle Eastern couple introduced themselves during my consulting hours at the university hospital. Neither of them spoke German or English, so they'd brought with them an interpreter, whose language skills were only slightly better than their own. And there we sat, we four, staring in silence at the spermiogram they'd brought from their home country.

The three in front of my desk were certainly somewhat unsettled by my mistrustful facial expression, but eventually, even with huge effort, I couldn't hide an incredulous smile—not with the information that was in front of me. How on earth was it possible that with 280 million sperm per milliliter—which is a hell of a lot—all 280 million of the little swimmers were dead?

The lab and ultrasound results were so unremarkable that the search for the causes of childlessness, in view of the language barrier, would be difficult—and that is exactly what it proved it be.

Even after a simple question the consulting room would fill for a couple of minutes with heated discussions, which from my point of view could just as easily have been about camels and curved knives, and what was being discussed was not the answer to the question that I had actually asked about, say, what medications the man regularly took. The interpreter did his best, but still the files of patients waiting for their appointments began to pile up on my desk.

Toward the end of the consultation, after we had excluded participation in an atom bomb test program and longtime drug addiction, I was at my wits' end. Then the head-scarfed wife, for the first time since entering my consulting room, indicated that she wanted to say something to me. Her husband and the interpreter tried to brush her aside, but people grasping at straws have to take chances, even if it means upsetting a man. So I asked the shy interpreter for a translation. The woman wanted to know whether it was normal that her husband bathed in boiling hot water several times a day.

"No, it's not," I replied, glancing at the patient with baffled severity. When I asked him to explain the reasons behind his unusual behavior, he sent his wife outside.

Now, in a male tête-à-tête-à-tête, he told me about his one and only affair. Allah had then plagued him with pains and a whitish discharge. So: a dose of clap. And as he couldn't go to a doctor in his home country, he thought he would use the power of water. Since then, he'd taken five steaming hot baths a day. *Eureka!* I thought. *He's been stewing his plums.* His wife was invited back to the circle and we spoke about treatment options.

"Antibiotics and a bathtub ban," I said. After four to six months, the two half-cooked sperm producers should have recovered. Again the *a*'s and *l*'s echoed around the room and the interpreter asked me in his inimitable German about the possibility of artificial insemination: "Husband ask why you not put sperm into egg of wife and then put both back in wife. Then you have baby in belly of wife."

My point that this procedure would be futile with dead sperm, and on top of that complex and expensive and anyway there were relatively good prospects of self-healing—as long as hot baths were avoided—didn't interest them. "Make sperm of husband in egg cell of wife, then baby in belly of wife," the interpreter said, persistently repeating the patients' wishes. In the meantime almost an hour had passed, and I began to rock uneasily on my stool. My next attempt at explaining that there could be no pregnancy using dead sperm for artificial insemination was equally unsuccessful. After the interpreter once more tried, mantra-like, to whine on about the principles of intracytoplasmic sperm injection in artificial insemination, I raised a hand to order a stop, eyed the audience seriously, and began with a spontaneous but thoroughly effective analogy.

"You can sit a dead bus driver in the driving seat of a bus, but it still won't move." The three looked at each other. A quick nod. Mission accomplished. Roughly a year and a half later, the couple produced a son.

LAB TESTING

A few words about microscopy. I no longer carry out spermiograms myself, as many patients simply couldn't afford to pay for them. Besides, the technicians in our lab are so good and experienced that I couldn't compete with them. Evaluating a spermiogram is absolute hell for beginners. People who've observed love juice under a microscope either become dizzy or feel as if they have a speeded-up bird's-eye view of a circus tent. Imagine treading on an anthill, focusing a camera on it, and having to count *which* ant is running when, where, and how fast! Chop-chop! The boss is waiting! We regularly have the quality of our tests certified in a sophisticated process in Münster, the mecca of European spermatology. Only then is it guaranteed that a lab really knows what it's doing. Our staff's training is long and pretty expensive, but it's worth it when the diagnostic results are correspondingly accurate.

Unfortunately, people often present me with spermiograms that indicate that the testing labs haven't invested in this level of quality training. Sometimes the measurements are inconclusive; sometimes certain results are missing entirely. In rare cases I'm presented with nothing but a handwritten note with "infertile" scrawled on it. So before going for a spermiogram, find out whether the lab participates in ring trials for quality control. After all, you don't go to a butcher to have your brakes tested.

Women's Fertility

OFTEN PATIENTS COME to our practice with their female partners to talk about their infertility. I'm certainly no gynecologist, and although the same hormones are present in both sexes, the female hormone system is far more complicated. However, I do like to ask a woman a few questions so I have as complete a picture of the couple's situation as possible. Mostly the women tell me, "My gynecologist said everything's okay."

On closer questioning, it often becomes apparent that the gynecologist wasn't making a diagnosis of the absence of pregnancy, but rather that the "everything's okay" referred to the gynecological state of the woman's health after her previous visit, when she was prescribed the pill. An ultrasound should, of course, be part of testing a woman's procreative capacity. On top of this, it can be important to carefully monitor her menstrual cycle, and thus her fertility cycle. A woman is not a hormonal atomic clock permanently ticking the same beat. Cycle variations of one to two weeks are not uncommon. This means that the fertile phase can also change and that it shouldn't be calculated from the beginning of the cycle but from the end. Often women show me the phone apps they use to calculate their fertile days. Unfortunately, all women's hormonal cycles and app software cannot be lumped together in a single equation. The results of these small mathematical aids are as helpful as saying that fish live in the sea, considering the diversity of species in the oceans.

A more precise method to find out the fertile days is to regularly measure body temperature. The day with the highest probability of a pregnancy is the day before ovulation. On the day of ovulation, a woman's morning temperature reading goes up by as much as 1 degree Fahrenheit (0.6 degrees Celsius). There isn't plenty of time left then for getting pregnant, as the day *after* ovulation the fertile phase is over. The egg cell survives only about twenty-four hours after ovulation, though sperm can swim around in the uterus and fallopian tubes for up to five days looking for the released egg.

There are other ways of determining women's fertile days. During the infertile phase of the cycle, viscous mucus forms at the cervix (the neck of the uterus), which, due to its consistency and chemical makeup, prevents sperm from infiltrating. In the fertile five or so days leading up to ovulation, as the body prepares itself for a potential pregnancy, the cervical mucus transforms: it becomes clear and no longer sticky to the touch (low viscosity). Then, after ovulation, the mucus becomes sticky again. The cervical mucus's chemistry changes during the fertile phase too, through the release of estrogen, resulting in an increase in minerals and glucose and a decline in acidity. Women's estrogen levels during the fertile phase ensure that sperm feel good in this environment, have enough energy, and are given access to the egg cell in the first place.

People who are having trouble coping with the temperature method or with gauging cervical mucus or who have failed to get consistent results can fall back on somewhat more expensive but more precise alternatives. Most drug stores sell test sticks that register the amounts of specific hormones in morning urine. Depending on the goal—contraception or pregnancy—there are various options that measure different hormone levels to provide the needed information. These findings are also not cast iron, but do provide a certain amount of security in determining the fertile days.

The *most* precise method to establish the timing of ovulation is ultrasound examination of the ovaries. In the development of the egg cell, the growth of the ovarian follicle is clearly visible with ultrasound. When the egg is released, the ovarian follicle collapses. This too appears on ultrasound scans.

Once the timing of ovulation has been established and if a woman's cycle is regular, the date of the next ovulation can be calculated with a fair degree of certainty, so that people wanting children can concentrate on the fertile phases. Having said that, a number of factors—stress, illness, parties, alcohol, jet lag, and sleep deprivation, to name but a few—can cause fluctuations in hormonal processes leading to irregularities so that ovulation doesn't occur as punctually as expected or hoped for.

When looking for causes for the failure of pregnancy, besides the typical pregnancy hormones, you should keep an eye on thyroid hormones. The thyroid glands, as the primary hormone-producing organ, have a watchdog function, making sure that all the other hormonal processes in the body are doing what they are supposed to be doing. Pregnancy in a woman is hormonal party time, so the thyroid should be in good working order. The general functions of the thyroid can be evaluated by testing the thyroid-stimulating hormone (TSH), a control hormone produced by the anterior pituitary gland. As long as we're considering the thyroid only, values below 3.5 nanograms per milliliter are good enough. (Depending on the measurement method, the upper threshold can be as high as 5.5 nanograms per milliliter.) For women who are trying to get pregnant, a number of scientific studies have shown that TSH values of 1 and lower are associated with considerably higher chances of pregnancy. The lower the TSH values, the more active the thyroid functions, so a lower number shows that higher amounts of active thyroid hormones are in the bloodstream. This is why even with normal TSH levels, say, 2.7, it's useful to take thyroid hormone pills.

Treatment Options: Sperm Meets Egg

WHEN THE MENSTRUAL cycle is ticking like a Rolex, the egg gamboling like Nureyev, and an army of Usain Bolts darting around but still there is no pregnancy, then maybe ways should be found to make sure that the sperm can find the egg. If you're planning to move to Key West and the bridge is closed, you aren't going to make your move-in date. If the fallopian tubes—the link between the ovaries and the uterus—are impermeable, there will be no pregnancy, regardless of how well the eggs and sperm are functioning.

The aftereffects of a chlamydia infection or endometriosis (in which portions of the uterus's mucous membrane obstruct the fallopian tubes) often include clogged fallopian tubes. Gynecological operations or adhesions in the abdomen can also affect passage through the tubes. The openness of the fallopian tubes can be checked using two different methods. For the first, an ultrasound of the uterus, blue dye is injected in both fallopian tubes. At the same time, a laparoscopy is performed, in which a fiber-optic camera is fed through the navel into the abdomen to monitor the blue dye's exit at the other end of the fallopian tubes. The patient requires a full anesthetic, and in very rare cases injuries arise when inserting the camera. The advantage of this method is that you can make very precise judgments about the situation inside the abdomen. On top of this, sometimes obstructions or adhesions can be removed during the examination to open the passage through the tubes. Other diagnoses can be discovered during a laparoscopy that hadn't been considered previously.

The second method of checking the openness of the fallopian tubes, requiring no general anesthetic or laparoscopy, has been known for a while but unfortunately is not used all that often. In this method, we use a syringe and a tube to pump a little air into the fallopian tubes. Normally, there's no air in the abdomen or in the region of the ovaries. Air fundamentally disturbs the ultrasound examination process. If air is pumped from the uterus into the fallopian tubes and the ultrasound scan of the ovaries displays typical disturbances—then voilà! There are no obstacles in the tubes.

If the woman still doesn't become pregnant, there are, finally, three different approaches to support pregnancy.

The first is artificial insemination, in which, using a catheter, sperm is injected in the direct vicinity of the opening of the fallopian tubes in the uterus, usually on the day before ovulation. The timing has to be carefully chosen so that the sperm is spared the journey from the cervix to somewhere way up the fallopian tubes, where sperm usually encounters the egg released from the ovary. It's a bit like carrying your dog to the dog park, but sometimes it helps. There are a few preconditions to fulfill for this simple method to work. You don't need a Ferrari of a spermiogram for artificial insemination to succeed, but you do need a certain sperm count. And the sperm have to be mobile. The long trip to the egg cell has indeed been artificially shortened, but still, penetration of the egg cell is only possible with active sperm movement. The spermiogram measurements that are required before the procedure will be done vary from practitioner to practitioner. An advantage of this method is that it can be carried out repeatedly at reasonably low costs. A woman also doesn't have to be pretreated with large quantities of hormones, as is the case in the next methods. The disadvantages are that the chances of success are not really impressive and a certain quality of sperm must be available before even considering this approach.

The remaining two methods of artificial insemination are considerably more complex, especially for the woman. In vitro fertilization (IVF) and intracytoplasmic sperm injection (ICSI) involve, first of all, hormonal stimulation of the woman in order to be able to harvest enough egg cells. It sounds about as romantic as it is. High doses of hormones drive the ovaries into the red light range and induce the development of multiple ovary follicles. The egg cells are retrieved using aspiration with an ultrasound-guided needle, then prepared for further treatment.

For IVF the man's sperm is incubated together with an egg cell in a test tube, the object being a natural fertilization *outside* the body. A few days later, at the onset of the cleavage stage, when the egg begins to divide, the embryo is transferred to the uterus. For ICSI a single sperm is selected under a microscope and injected into the egg cell. Here too there is artificial insemination outside the body, and here too after a few days the egg cell is replanted in the uterus after the egg has begun to divide in the incubator. IVF requires a certain amount of sperm with good motility. But fertility centers like to perform ICSI even when sperm parameters are in fact sufficient for IVF. In my opinion IVF, even with all the support measures, allows life somehow to find its own way. With ICSI it is ultimately the embryologist at the microscope who chooses the sperm for fertilization. Hopefully, that person isn't having a bad day...

All these tests and treatments are carried out in highly specialized fertility clinics. If artificial insemination results in pregnancy and birth, then that's wonderful! The other side of the coin is that treatment is expensive, patients often have to pay at least part of the costs themselves, and success—the birth of a child—can be expected in considerably fewer than half the cases. This applies even to couples who don't seem to have any other health issues. As a normal pregnancy can happen in a couple of years, I view the involvement of fertility clinics somewhat critically, especially where young couples are concerned. From time to time you get the impression that men at these clinics are there only as suppliers of sperm. Whether the sperm is good or bad quality is ultimately not really that important, as ICSI can still be performed even with particularly bad spermiograms. Meanwhile, a thorough examination by an andrologist with treatment targeted at improving sperm quality is not always considered as an option. It's common that patients with poor spermiograms ask me for a second opinion after a couple of unsuccessful ICSIS. During these talks it regularly becomes apparent that not even ultrasounds were done by the fertility clinic, let alone specific lab tests. Undoubtedly, the fertility clinics do a good job, and of course highly specialized clinics have to be financially viable. It's just that I wish the man and *his* situation were given a bit more attention and that couples were given a little more time to have a natural pregnancy.

If all this is simply a "first-world" problem—after having a third son, you would like to have a daughter—here are some not particularly scientific tips. Evidence from history doesn't really support the theory that hot baths, testicle tourniquets, or right- or left-side positions during sexual intercourse result in the desired sex of offspring. A boy is conceived when X and Y chromosomes come together, and a girl when it's two X chromosomes. Egg cells, from mothers, always have an X chromosome; the sperm of fathers can contain an X or Y chromosome. So in the final analysis, it is men who determine whether a Martina or a Martin is about to arrive.

Ever since this was discovered, men have tried to influence the sex of their offspring. Socks, pepper, or a glass of gin before intercourse don't have a significant effect. Research has indicated that sperm with X chromosomes are slower movers but as compensation have more stamina. Sperm with Y chromosomes are quicker but have shorter lives. If ovulation is as regular as a Swiss watch, this information can be used in progeny planning. If intercourse occurs shortly before ovulation, the speedy male Y chromosome reaches the egg cell first and a boy is conceived. If intercourse takes place three or four days before ovulation, the already tired male Y chromosome sperm are out of the race, the X chromosome tortoise reaches the finishing line, and a girl is conceived. In 1991 a U.S. study was published showing that the results for six couples following these guidelines were at least "statistically significant." In this context, the Gralla family can also add some input. I'm one of three brothers, and then my mother conceived my sister, Carolin, using this method.

Finally, an example from my practice of how fertility treatment can work at the andrologist. A patient who had wanted children for a long time came to my practice. This wasn't any old patient but my oldest and still best friend. After sitting at school together, skipping math, and going on holiday together, it felt slightly odd to have him sitting in front of me during my consulting hours—above all, because the results of his tests were a spermatological disaster. What followed was a broadside from the whole spectrum of andrological therapy. Antibiotic treatment was initiated to counter various documented infections that are normally controlled microbiologically. Antiestrogen therapy was launched to stabilize testosterone levels and deal with testicle function problems caused by hormonal irregularities. High-dose orthomolecular treatment with various antioxidants specifically targeted his limited sperm motility because there were signs of oxidative stress. On top of that, Doppler-ultrasound scans led to a diagnosis of bilateral varicocele, which required laparoscopic surgery. Over the course of several appointments, we also talked about walking slightly differently, to improve his health in general.

Slowly but surely, his spermiograms began to record improvements. To our great satisfaction, after two years the spermiogram readings were within the normal range. But as I always say, "You don't want a good spermiogram on your lap—you want a child." The first son arrived a year later by means of ICSI. What happened next delighted me beyond measure. During paternity leave, my friend, his wife, and child decided to cross Australia in a camper. "Enjoying barbies every day, one or two beers, and spectacular sunsets" was the secret recipe. Their second son, conceived near Melbourne, is 7 years old as I write this.

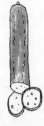

five

MALE CONTRACEPTION: REVERSE EQUALITY

CONTRACEPTION, DEPENDING ON your personal situation, is very sensible, and not only once the horde of diaper-destroying bawlers are beyond the first hurdle and you can dedicate your nights to catching up on some restful sleep. There are many contraceptive methods that you can more or less rely on so as not to have to add another extension to your house for yet another child's room. A number of these methods are based on the fact that the woman has to hazard her health in childbirth, or at the very least wants childbearing not to have a negative influence on the quality of her life.

The contraceptive pill, commonly referred to just as the pill—regardless of how well it works and how much it has changed women's self-determination—brings with it a heap of potential side effects. Here we're not talking about just a little fluid retention, invisible to her partner, that makes her favorite blouse a little bit tight at the waist. We're talking about anything from pathological changes to the cardiovascular system to heart attacks and strokes—although, thank goodness, only very rarely.

There are, however, where contraception is concerned, ways for men to take the initiative. The most common option is using the humble little sheath—a process supposedly inaugurated by a certain Dr. Condom (although verification of that has proved to be elusive)—in which, initially, dried sheep's gut was slipped over the love muscle. Casanova used this not particularly vegan contraceptive method to avoid syphilis, which was rampant in his day. After Charles Goodyear—yes, the tire man—developed vulcanized rubber, the first rubber condoms began appearing on the market in the 1850s, and the musty sheep's gut understandably became history. In about 1920 latex condoms were developed, which looked less like bike inner tubes and thus introduced a bit of fun into the act. In the ensuing decades the ideas of the producers were only limited by the bounds of imagination, so nowadays there are condoms in flavors that would wrinkle the brow of a fruit seller at the farmers' market, condoms that reduce the likelihood of a premature ejaculation, and even condoms that improve the stiffness of an erection! Beware of using cooking oil as a lubricant—some members of the American gay scene in the 1970s liked to use this inexpensive and neutral smelling Vaseline surrogate without realizing that oil-based lubes attack latex, causing it to split, so that men on practicing their occasionally athletic skills were confronted with exploding condoms flying all over the place.

A somewhat more drastic method of avoiding unwanted offspring was practiced in Rome centuries ago. It involved dipping the family jewels in piping hot water, which made the decision about whether it would be a Tony or a Cleo redundant for a couple of months. While the sheep's gut/vulcanized rubber/latex condom was able to become a fixed feature of every wallet and nightstand drawer of copulating couples, adherents of the "boiled balls" family planning faction still lead a shadowy existence on the internet and even in my practice. In fifteen years, only one of these undaunted gonad scorchers has strayed into my office, but he managed to ask me, with a deadpan expression, whether it had to be forty-five minutes at 50 degrees (Celsius, not Fahrenheit!) or whether sixty minutes at 45 degrees would be sufficient to save money on diapers. Somewhat bewildered but remaining friendly, I explained to him that I had training as neither a chef nor a baker, and that for cooking I still had to refer to a recipe book. Alternatively, he could simply place his balls on a conveniently high kitchen work surface and give them a couple of deft whacks with a meat mallet or a thick cookbook. It's faster and would have the same effect. If necessary, a Bible could be used instead of the cookbook—maybe then there would be an expression of approval from the Vatican.

If, however, a man is looking for a safe, almost painless, and also reversible method to spare himself an heir and not to have to dangle a hairy scrotum in a humiliating position above a steaming hot cauldron while anticipating the excruciating agony, then there's always a vasectomy.

Snip: The Vasectomy

A VASECTOMY IS a surgical procedure for men in which both sides of the vas deferens are severed, preventing sperm from the testicles from reaching open air or, as the case may be, the uterus of the partner. As I insist during consultations, "EVERYTHING—ELSE—REMAINS—THE—SAME!" This applies to erection capability, the libido, hormone levels, ejaculation, and the quality of orgasms. The erection, as I have pointed out, depends on many things, but ultimately on the influx of blood into the cavernous body. Sperm have nothing—but absolutely nothing—to do with it. It's true that testicles produce testosterone, which is sometimes crucial to the libido, and without libido, no erection, but testosterone is distributed by the bloodstream, whereas sperm are transported from the testicles by the vas deferens. They won't be after the operation, but still, there are no changes to the ability to achieve an erection.

People often give me a funny look when I tell them that there are also no significant changes in ejaculation. Most of the volume of the ejaculate comes from the prostate and the seminal vesicles, and contains plenty of nourishment for sperm so that the tiny rascals don't founder on the way to the egg cell. This—over 90 percent of the volume of ejaculate—remains after the operation and, depending on the strength of the pelvic floor, erupts on ejaculation at an average speed of almost 30 miles per hour and can travel almost 20 feet (that's 6 meters at 45 kilometers per hour). World record! The orgasm also remains as it was—a neural firework display in pelvis and head not least invoked by the whoosh of ejaculation shooting through the urethra, creating a sexual shock wave throughout the organ well supplied with plenty of nerve cells.

The major advantages of a vasectomy are obvious. The operation—it takes ten minutes under a local anesthetic, and we always play music and have a nice chat with the patient—is the safest form of contraception there is. The effectiveness of a birth control method is measured on the Pearl Index. This scale registers the number of pregnancies that happen despite a man or woman following one form or other of contraception. On the index, vasectomy registers 0.1 (0.1 percent contraceptive failure), the pill up to 1, and condoms between 2 and 20. The contraceptive practices of our above-mentioned ballsack boiler have yet to be listed on the index but are probably well above body temperature.

Changing Your Mind: Vasectomy Reversal

ALSO NOT TO be forgotten: a vasectomy is reversible. The reversal operation is considerably more complex, but in the hands of an experienced surgeon success rates are well over 90 percent. I used to carry out these operations, and they're pretty enthralling. Picture this: You saw cleanly through a matchstick—the vas deferens is roughly that thick. At each of the cut edges, you make tiny holes in the wood with a fine needle. These two holes represent the passageway of the inside of the vas deferens and have to be sewn together during the operation. For the operation to succeed, you (the surgeon) should seriously consider the amount of alcohol you drink the evening before and the number of cups of coffee you treat yourself to at breakfast.

In Germany, some 55,000 men have a vasectomy annually, and the trend is rising sharply—about 500,000 in the United States. Depending on which clinical study you read, 3 to 6 percent of vasectomies are later reversed by vasovasostomy. The reasons are diverse. Very often a man has separated from his partner and, in a new relationship, his desire for children has been reawakened. Less commonly, a couple had, earlier, conceived a child while not really wanting one and had decided on a vasectomy before it happened again. Once their relationship has become stable and their professional or social circumstances have settled, they can, with a vasovasostomy, resume planning a larger family. A sad reason for a refertilization operation is the death of a child, after which the couple again want offspring. All, I think, are absolutely legitimate reasons.

If you bear in mind the time span between vasectomy and reversal—on average some eight years—and call upon your high school math skills, you can calculate what the pill would have cost instead. A vasectomy, in Germany, costs somewhere between 400 and 600 euros (US$450 to $700—reversal is about five times that). For eight years of the pill, including acne, fluid retention, and cardiovascular risks, a German woman would have to pay almost 1,000 euros (over US$1,000) and, as already stated, the dependability of hormonal contraception is considerably less than that of a vasectomy. (In the U.S., a vasectomy costs up to $1,000, and eight years of the pill anywhere from $800 to $8,000, depending on what's prescribed. In some Canadian provinces, vasectomies are covered by public health insurance, while eight years on the pill adds up to about $2,000.)

The fact that reversing the operation, even after years or decades, can pay off is witnessed by gentlemen such as Charlie Chaplin, Anthony Quinn, and Mick Jagger, who, in their seventies, were again able to relish the joys of fatherhood. Advanced age for men is not the hurdle it is for women. Scientific papers on vasovasostomy regularly report that ten years after a vasectomy, sperm production is thought to decrease considerably due to long-term pressure on the testicular tissues. But I've operated on patients daring to make the step toward family planning *twenty* years after their initial operation, and even after such a long time the refertilization operation still made sense. In the course of reversal surgery, a smear is taken from the part of the vas deferens that comes from the testicles. While we're still in the operating theater, the smear is analyzed under a microscope for sperm cells. If the findings are positive, then, depending on the skills of the surgeon, (almost) nothing should stand in the way of fatherhood.

Sperm production often requires a certain amount of time to recover, so people shouldn't reckon on an immediate pregnancy. After surgery, some time should pass before attempting to fulfill the desire for children. Overly eager men who, as soon as they wake up from the anesthetic, want to get down to business—even in the hospital parking lot—would be well advised to take their time if they don't want the freshly sewn tubes to burst. Wait two or three weeks and the anastomosis, the new connection, will hold.

A check on the success of the operation, in the form of a postoperative spermiogram, should be made within a couple of months. If live sperm are found, then the operation was a success.

Naturally, even after successful surgery and proof of living sperm, it's still possible that a pregnancy won't occur. First, a normal spermiogram for a man who has just had surgery obviously doesn't mean that everything is okay for his partner. What's more, after a vasectomy some patients suffer from immunological reactions that put a stop to pregnancy by normal means. In my practice it's not unusual for patients, especially after vasectomy reversals, to have positive MAR tests in the spermiogram. MAR here doesn't refer to the Mid-Atlantic Ridge or a micro assault rifle, as some people might think, but to a *mixed antiglobulin reaction*.

The MAR test checks whether the man who owns the testicles from which the sperm that is wriggling under the microscope originated has produced antibodies *against* his own sperm. It is indeed unfortunate, but it happens. If there have been microscopic injuries to blood vessels in the testicles—from an operation, inflammations, or other injuries—the blood–testis barrier is disrupted. This is not the border crossing between the countries of Blood and Testis but the internal lining of blood vessels in the testicular tissue. The interior walls of the blood vessels here are virtually complete and fully wallpapered. In other parts of the body, the internal linings are fenestrated, meaning that there are small gaps (like windows) enabling exchange with cells or proteins from the surrounding tissues. Not so with (healthy) testicles! The reason for this is that sperm have a different set of chromosomes to other body cells. Sperm are, so to speak, only half human and need to be fused with a female egg cell to become a complete building block. In this respect sperm in the body are foreign matter that belongs behind bars, or, in this case, behind the blood–testis barrier. If in some way this barrier is damaged, then sperm are in direct contact with the body's police force—the immune cells, who, on swimming up to the sperm, recognize them as strangers: "Your identification, please…" What does a healthy immune system do on identifying a foreign body? That's right: it produces antibodies to prevent something worse from happening. The problem is that, as in real life, sometimes the innocent end up behind bars. With sperm the equivalent problem is that the antibodies on the sperm mean that the tiny swimmers can no longer continue moving in the woman's uterus. The woman's decidua—the lining of the uterus—is coated on the surface with antigens which, together with the antibodies on the sperm, cause an antigen-antibody reaction with an effect something like a zipper. Sperm congregating in the uterus become entangled with each other and remain on the spot, wriggling around like a pack of dogs on a dogwalker's leash. They can't even have a go at the mail carrier.

The MAR test imitates this behavior. A special antiserum with tiny latex particles is mixed with the ejaculate. If the sperm contains antibodies, it will react to the serum. Without the latex beads, the sperm can be seen under a microscope, racing around; with the tiny beads, the sperm with antibodies tack onto them and wriggle around on the spot. One hundred sperm specimens are counted out, and if more than fifty are attached to the beads, then the test is positive and the patient is considered immunologically infertile. At least that's what the textbooks say. In my practice I've had a number of patients who, despite testing positive in the MAR tests, have produced a child. This is understandable if we again call on our high school math. Assume a man produces 200 million sperm, 60 percent of which become attracted to the latex beads during the MAR test, resulting in a positive result (which, counterintuitively, means "infertile"). Mathematically this still means that 40 percent—80 million sperm—are free of antibodies. For a normal spermiogram, you need 39 million sperm, so just less than half. Why then, according to the textbooks, is this immunological infertility? I can't tell you. It's possible that the situation continues to evolve and in the course of a few months the number of positive sperm in the MAR test increases. Perhaps the sperm that didn't register positive in the test were subject to immunological reactions that didn't appear under laboratory conditions.

But even with a positive MAR test, it's not the end of the world. The results of these tests are not cast iron; a follow-up test should be performed after three months. If that is also positive, low-dose naltrexone therapy could be tried. This involves taking a small dose of opioid protagonists at night. High doses make alcohol withdrawal symptoms tolerable; low doses (specifically at night) modulate the immune system, and sperm autoantibodies disperse. Unfortunately, there hasn't been a study supporting this, but it has worked plenty of times in practice. Long live off-label therapy! If, over a long period of time, the antibodies don't disappear and the attempt at low-dose therapy fails, then you are the perfect patient for ICSI treatment, with optimal pregnancy outcomes.

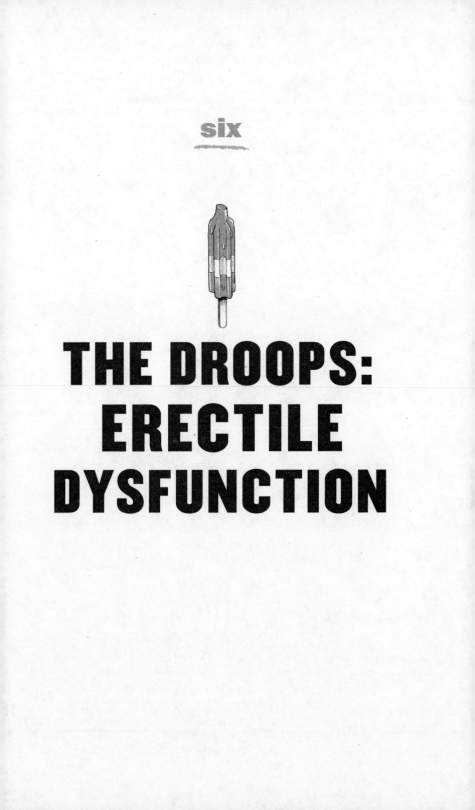

six

THE DROOPS: ERECTILE DYSFUNCTION

E RECTION FAILURE—OR as the pros say, erectile dysfunction, often shortened to ED—can occur at any age. According to the largest scientific study on the subject, which questioned and examined thousands of patients, ED is more frequent in the older age range. The rule of thumb is 70 percent of 70-year-olds. However, I've discovered that there are apparently some exceptional retirees.

In my very first week as a urologist, I was confronted face to face with the topic of sexuality and old age. Mr. M. was a ripe old 96-year-old and, with all due respect, he didn't look a day younger. Two world wars had left their marks on his outward appearance. One arm was missing, and the other held a crutch to help him walk—the "fucking Russians," who usually used only dud hand grenades, had used a live one, which, on being thrown back, had exploded, embedding shrapnel in Mr. M. and forever scarring the vibrant veteran's face. One eye had been replaced by a slightly fanciful glass one.

He came to us with a small ulceration on his foreskin that bled from time to time. After noting down his medical history and taking blood samples, I led the elderly gentleman, who was somewhat wobbly on his legs, into my examination room and discovered the odd war wound but nothing more serious. Finally I explained to the patient the operation, the risks, and the possible complications. After having signed the consent form, he inquired, "And what about getting a license to ride after the operation?"

Doctors don't generally approve of any kind of driving for patients his age and use their powers to try to dissuade them from venturing onto the roads. But the gentleman was exceptionally likable and I was interested in his countless stays in field hospitals in both world wars, and those things plus the fact that he had reached an almost biblical age must have softened my resolve. "Yes, okay," I said. "You can apply for a motorcycle license."

The old man looked at me irritably. "Motorcycle license? What motorcycle? What on earth are you talking about?" Rather defensively, I replied with an apprehensive smile, "Well, you did ask me about riding. What did you mean?"

"What do you think? Not *biking* riding but *bonking* riding, of course! How long do I have to wait after the operation before I can have sex again?"

I learned that day that a rousing lust for life has nothing to do with age.

When Is ED ED—and When Is a Man a Man?

THE YOUNGEST PATIENT I've ever had with ED had just turned 14—which raises the first question: When is erectile dysfunction erectile dysfunction, or rather, what is actually "normal"? The medical definition is: When satisfactory sexual intercourse has not been possible for more than two months. This is not just a funny definition for laypeople, and it raises a whole series of questions. For instance: "How often have you been tempted to have sex in the last few months?" and "What exactly is satisfactory intercourse?" Ultimately, people's natures are different, and no harm is done by doctors and patients agreeing on the common ground—or you end up with a case like this...

The young man had obviously summoned up all his courage and, with large, inquiring eyes and a slight stutter, he revealed the purpose of his visit: "Doctor Gralla, er... There's something wrong with my erection..." After I asked him what exactly was wrong with his erection, he disclosed remorsefully that he had managed to give his girlfriend only two orgasms and at the third attempt it just hadn't happened, adding that this couldn't possibly be normal. At 14! My astonishment grew as it became apparent that he had already found the diagnosis and, as a fresh ex-virgin teenager, had made an appointment to see me. Nipping things in the bud, as it were. The question arises, Where and how on earth do the kids of today get to know their sexuality? I am firmly convinced that internet portals like YouPorn have led kids to believe in a hypersexualized world. Putting it bluntly, nowadays all kinds of fetishes can be indulged in by watching hundreds of clips on your phone without your parents having the faintest idea what's happening. And when a young man's first love doesn't wear a double-D bra, isn't coffee colored and mightily sexy, then a short-term case of the droops becomes a relationship crisis or worse.

I didn't prescribe this young kid any medication, but rather advised him to give himself and his girlfriend a bit of time and not to waste his pocket money on Viagra.

Four Reasons for the Droops

ALTHOUGH THE BOY'S problem had more to do with physical excess and lack of self-esteem, there are, of course, patients who really *do* suffer from erectile dysfunction. There are many reasons for the "droops." I divide the most common causes into four groups: organs, toxins, hormones, and the psyche.

ORGANS

Organic causes of erectile dysfunction include everything that incapacitates the actual functioning of the cavernous body.

During an erection, blood flows through arteries in the middle of the penile tissues, which absorb the blood like a sponge. The walls of the cavernous body are pretty durable, and at some stage the tissues are so full that the pressure in the penis increases considerably. By means of this pressure, the flow of blood to the outer reaches of the penile tissues, where the drainage system is located, is squeezed nearly shut. If this ultimately mechanical but still intricate

interlinkage between allowing an influx of blood and preventing it from draining is impaired by dysfunctional blood
vessels, the result is what is sometimes termed, rather flip-
pantly, the droops. This disorder can be either arterial, from
the inflowing blood system, or venous, from the outflowing
blood system. It's often caused by high blood pressure, diabetes, arteriosclerosis, neurological or metabolic disorders,
smoking, or any number of other diseases that damage
blood vessels or their functions.

As to things that can happen to that blood flow...

Herbert B. ended up in Emergency, and the attending
doctor, looking slightly irritated, was given the following
explanation of why. On this particular day at work, there
was nothing much to do and Mr. B. really felt the urge to do
something of a sexual nature, so he made the bold decision
to satisfy his physical needs. He looked to his surroundings—he worked in a mechanic's shop—for inspiration.
As his age was exacting its toll—he was about 50 and no
longer had boundless confidence in the powers of his erection—he slipped 4-millimeter-thick ring washers (about
⅛ inch), which, according to him, are used in the bridge
building industry, over his penis. Not one or two—no, he
settled on *three* of these mechanical aids, possibly on the
assumption that two couldn't possibly withstand the force
of his erection. They quickly took effect and, probably in
front of a pinup calendar, the man was bestowed with a fine,
eyebrow-raising erection.

Normally, and for good reason, penis rings are made to
be removed after their intended effect has been fulfilled, so
that the blood from the aroused penis can circulate again.

This is not the case for thick industrial steel ring washers. When after an hour, the washers still firmly in situ, the pink of his pride and joy began to acquire the color of an eggplant and the pain became unbearable, the man made his second fateful, but this time correct, decision: the washers had to go—and quickly! Full of drive and with a fully erect penis, he rummaged through the shelves and chanced upon a small electric-powered tool onto which a wide range of attachments could be affixed to accomplish any number of the tasks at hand—polishing, grinding, sanding, drilling, sawing...

After a good two hours Mr. B. had managed to open one of the three washers, at least partially, but he had to abandon the project because as an experienced mechanic, he realized that cutting through thick bridge-building steel washers and removing them are two different things. With frayed nerves and DayGlo eggplant-colored penis, he laid down his arms and resolved to visit the pros.

On inspecting the thing projecting from between his legs, you could only vaguely guess how many times the small screeching saw must have slipped, the heat that must have been generated during this torture, and how much Mr. B. must have hated himself for his carnal curiosity, especially as the next day there was to be a large family gathering for the baptism of his granddaughter.

By now his penis wasn't only the color of an eggplant but also the dimensions of one, albeit one for which a hobby gardener would have run away with first prize at a vegetable show.

After a cursory assessment, the senior duty physician sullenly eyed the patient with the disfigured member, emitting no more than occasional staccato-like hmmms, and ordered an anesthetic.

Although for urologists it would be considered a heavy-duty piece of equipment, the tool that the instrument nurse handed over from the orthopedic instrument tray couldn't remove even the washer that the patient had so painstakingly managed to break. After two or three more or less delicate attempts, the experienced senior physician began to lose patience: "Oh, shit! This is getting us nowhere—we need some *proper* equipment." The janitor was informed and brought a giant pair of bolt cutters, the type that sever the locks of illegally parked bikes.

After hesitant positioning of this terrifying instrument and constant repositioning in an attempt to cause as little damage as possible, the doctor, without thinking of keeping his voice down, spluttered an irritated "It really doesn't matter anymore" and with great exertion, brought the two blades together. As if he had severed an overstrung piano string with a pair of nail scissors, there came the high metallic *ping* of the first washer flying through the air, landing on the floor like a tossed coin, and spinning to a standstill beneath the sink.

You could literally sense the smug smile of satisfaction spreading across the doctor's face beneath his green surgical mask even while the sound of the dancing washer was echoing around the theater. *Behold! I have conquered industrial steel!*

With the same technique, the other two washers were removed without further problems, and the penis now resembled the flesh-colored remnants of some lathe work that hadn't been particularly well executed. Warmly wrapped in bandages and smeared with all the ointments that could be found, Mr. B. was finally taken to the ward, where everybody was eagerly awaiting him.

After a week, with his private parts now resembling a large pickled cucumber in both size and color, Mr. B. was released from hospital. He had, however, missed the baptism.

TOXINS

Besides organic causes, there are medicinal (and toxic, or poisonous) triggers of ED. Many medications, particularly those treating the cardiovascular system and metabolic diseases, cause erectile dysfunction as a side effect. This makes it sound as if you are jumping from the frying pan into the fire. However, when a patient is admitted to hospital moving robotically, with a blood pressure crisis and a face the color of a beet, then planning a romantic weekend with his partner is slightly lower down on the priority list for the time being. The primary concern of doctors in Emergency in such cases is (hopefully!) the patient's physical welfare. They don't intend to put certain body parts to sleep—that's a side effect of medication.

Beta blockers, for instance—but also other drugs used in lowering blood pressure—are not exactly conducive to erections. People prescribed sartans (angiotensin receptor blockers), however, can be grateful to their GP, internist, or cardiologist, as these drugs have no damaging effect on erections. And if it *has* to be a beta blocker, then you can hope for the one that is least damaging—nebivolol. However, all kinds of psychiatric, anti-allergen, and even antifungal medications can spoil a healthy erection.

TESTOSTERONE

Hormonal disorders can also be the cause of erectile dysfunction. The main male hormone, quite simply, is testosterone. The juggernaut of all sexual hormones has a chapter dedicated to it later, but it deserves a book. The thyroid glands and the associated hormones are also not unimportant to men, but they are very seldom the causes of erectile dysfunctions.

KNOTS IN THE HEAD: THE DEAR OLD PSYCHE

Few men can get used to the idea of suffering from a psychosomatic disorder. After all, they don't have any screws loose—it just doesn't do what it's supposed to do. If the door hinges jam, you go to the hardware store and buy replacements. Thoughts are similar about erectile dysfunctions, preferably something crisply organic that can be corrected with a few pills or some ointment. Still, psychosomatic causes are more common than you imagine.

There are many possible explanations for sexual knots in the head. Sometimes the causes are literally way back in childhood. Often a previous partner is involved. Sometimes the current relationship is too perfect or too familiar. Just think for a moment about how closely or how long you want to go through life with your partner.

After many years, the boundaries become blurred and in terms of feelings of familiarity, having sex with your partner is like having sex with a member of your family—subconsciously, of course. Often our expectations of ourselves are unrealistic. Sometimes our partner is too demanding. A great many things in and around sex can remain unspoken or unclear.

Ultimately, sex is a kind of individual togetherness and you could be rightly astonished that it ever works at the drop of a hat. You should be allowed a few attempts before you know which buttons to press for sex to be a pleasure for both parties. In this respect, women have a far greater range of buttons than men. A colleague summed things up succinctly: men are like toasters, women like accordions.

Getting Things Rolling Again

AFTER OPEN DISCUSSIONS between patient and doctor (which can alone make a huge contribution) and arriving at a diagnosis, the appropriate form of treatment has to be decided upon. Sometimes I find that it helps to simply glance at the birthdate of the patient sitting on the other side of the desk. A 25-year-old athlete is unlikely to have diabetes or to be hauling around a massive cholesterol problem. A lack of hormones is also unusual in someone his age. (Incidentally, after years in andrology you can spot a man with a testosterone deficiency as soon as he enters the room, but more on that later.) If no pharmaceutical erection-crushers have been taken, and recreational drugs have been excluded—alcohol, marijuana, cocaine, LSD, and the like are all prejudicial to a healthy erection in the long term!—then all that remains is the dear old psyche.

During discussions of treatment options, I invariably recommend a psychological solution to a patient with a suspected psychosomatic ED. This doesn't necessarily mean popping round the corner to the nearest psychotherapist. Sexual therapy is a very wide field requiring special expertise but is, unfortunately, rarely covered by insurance. Depending on the problem, it can take eight to twelve sessions to unravel the knots. Many patients shy away from going to sexual therapists or can't afford to. There are, however, other ways of getting the sexual impulses rolling.

THE LITTLE BLUE PILL

Viagra arrived on the market in 1998 and revolutionized andrology, if not the whole field of sex. Medications before this time were full of unwanted side effects, and often enough we gave the old penis a jab of it, to no visible effect other than pain. With the arrival of the little blue pill, it was suddenly possible to perform real miracles and the side effects were mostly manageable. This was unimaginable previously—a medication designed for the long-term treatment of ED with organic causes, able to grant users a high quality of life. Today there are four different phosphodiesterase 5 (PDE5) inhibitors, which all seem to work and have earned their reputation.

The PDE5 inhibitors (Viagra, Cialis, Levitra, and Spedra) block the enzyme phosphodiesterase. PDE5 is present in high concentrations in the cavernous body of men, which is why the good targeted effects take place here.

After some intermediate stages, the inhibiting of enzymes finally results in prolonging or, as the case may be, improving the effects of nitrogen monoxide (NO, also known as nitric oxide). NO, in turn, expands blood vessels, allowing an increase in blood flow and thus improving men's ability to have an erection.

In my experience, even younger men with psychosomatic erectile dysfunctions can benefit from the drug, once they have been informed and are willing to try it. It's true that their blood vessels aren't pathologically affected, but still, a motor runs better on premium gas. With psychosomatic ED, involuntary impulses prevent relaxation of the vascular muscles in the penis and the increased influx of blood. Let me put it this way: if a Neandertal is standing in front of a saber-toothed tiger, he's not worrying about an erection—escape is the first thing on his mind, and an erection would be a great inconvenience. Not that the partner has to be a saber-toothed tiger. Stress (be it professional, interpersonal, bodily, financial, or any other such thing) and fear (especially fear of your own sexual failure) cause involuntary impulses that, in the end, support the primitive escape scenario.

For medicinal treatment of psychosomatic ED, I like to use an old medical trick: the patient begins with a high dosage but in lower individual amounts. This means that at the beginning of treatment the patient takes three to four low-dose pills more often to attain the corresponding high dose of the active ingredients. This should let him achieve a successful attempt at intercourse: the impressive dosage should release the involuntary brakes. Should it not work the first time, the second time with the same dosage is pretty certain to result in an erection that would do honor to even the most faint-hearted. Once self-confidence has been bolstered, then the next time the patient can concentrate on sex and his partner without being afraid that it won't work out, that the partner will be disappointed yet again, or that the problems will start all over.

Once you've broken through the negative barriers, the psyche can work to help, not hinder. At the next appointment, the dosage should be reduced by one pill, which for psychosomatic ED is almost always enough to attain an erection. I always advise patients to have sex a few times with the reduced dosage to regain sexual self-confidence with pharmaceutical support. Once sex has become relaxed and satisfactory, the dosage can again be lowered almost to a homeopathic maintenance dose, just enough to have some of the active ingredients in the bloodstream. The manufacturer's smallest recommended dosage can continue to be halved until use tapers off completely.

Some sexual therapists will probably throw up their hands in horror at this pragmatic strategy, but I maintain that sometimes the end justifies the means, especially when there's so much positive feedback—from both sexes. Before the therapy starts, it's important that I make clear that the dosage will be rigorously reduced to zero and that this is the only pack of pills I'll be prescribing him! With the correct dosage, the side effects are not dangerous, and it can improve the quality of life of a relationship as well as being a bit of fun. Nevertheless, in the long run these drugs *are* expensive for young people, and temporary knots in the head shouldn't make you dependent on the pharmaceutical industry.

ORTHOMOLECULAR OPTIONS

Besides PDE5 inhibitors, there are other options for getting an erection up and running. Orthomolecular therapy can be tried for mild cases of ED or in its early stages. Arginine is one of twenty amino acids that we absorb in our daily diets. It's present in pretty much everything that vegetarians and nonvegetarians eat—you'll find it in meats, nuts, and pumpkin seeds, for instance. Orthomolecular therapy means that supraphysiological doses—amounts greater than those normally found in the body—are administered to attain the desired results. This would mean at least a couple of bucketfuls of pumpkin seeds, which is why orthomolecular active ingredients are dispensed in a purer form, usually as powders or capsules.

L-arginine is an NO donor, meaning it's the only amino acid that transports nitrogen monoxide to the bloodstream. Nitrogen monoxide doesn't sound particularly sexy—more like suicide and car exhaust—but it's just the opposite. In 1988 there was even a Nobel Prize awarded for NO research, when Robert F. Furchgott and colleagues discovered what this molecule was capable of doing. Among other things, NO is a highly capable blood vessel expander, which incidentally, as we have seen, is also reflected in the mechanisms of the PDE5 inhibitors. Phosphodiesterase 5 speeds up the breakdown of NO. If the breakdown is inhibited, then more NO enters the bloodstream, triggering better erections. Importantly for Viagra and other associated drugs, type 5 of the phosphodiesterases is primarily urologic and found in particularly high concentrations in the cavernous body of the penis. L-arginine, on the other hand, passes on its NO anywhere. However, as various studies have shown, this is enough to improve an erection. Dosages should be around 6,000 milligrams a day, but the capsules available on the market are not to be recommended—who wants to swallow ten submarine-sized tablets a day? L-arginine is also available in powder form. It tastes disgusting, but mixed with pineapple juice, the flavor is hardly noticeable. There are other methods of taking L-arginine in dosages of up to 30,000 milligrams a day, and even at these concentrations you cannot overdose.

You could even take it a step further and try citrulline as an amino acid. Citrulline is present in high concentrations in watermelon rind and in the urea cycle as a precursor of L-arginine. The advantage is that it tastes a lot better than L-arginine and isn't metabolized as wastefully by the body, meaning that smaller doses are enough. The disadvantage is that up to now only one study has described its effects, and for us doctors, that's not enough.

EXPANDING SHOCK WAVES

Since 2011 there's been a newcomer to ED therapy, and this treatment method not only leads to an improvement in the symptoms but also restores or at least improves the prior status of the blood circulation in the cavernous body. During extracorporeal shock wave therapy (ESWT), the erectile tissue is bombarded by low-dose shock waves over a number of sessions, and although this sounds somewhat martial, it's absolutely painless. The shock wave impulses stimulate the growth of new blood vessels in the tissue.

A number of studies in recent years have shown that this therapy boosts circulation in the penis, allowing measurable improvements to the erection capacities. Dermatologists and surgeons use the same principle when treating patients with wound-healing disorders: ESWT encourages new blood vessels in the area of the wound, which greatly enhances the healing processes. All this becomes really exciting if we call on Furchgott's discovery. NO doesn't help only by expanding blood vessels but also by initiating the formation of new blood vessels in a variety of processes in the body such as wound healing, growth, and the development of the embryo in the womb. In our practice, ESWT is carried out in conjunction with doses of L-arginine to support the formation of new blood vessels from both directions.

... OR DIY

Other options for improving the erection capacities include therapies that have been practiced for a long time and that sometimes have good effects but whose execution is way down on the enjoyment scale. In medicated urethral system for erection therapy (MUSE) you have to feed a small plastic tube about an inch into the urethra to deposit a tablet the size of a grain of rice. After the tube has been withdrawn, the urethra is massaged from the outside so that the medication is absorbed into the cavernous body. Sometimes the procedure is successful, but it's often painful. And if things don't work out so well, the urethra begins to bleed which, in the long run, can lead to lesions. Alternatively, a gel can be used that, with a booster, is absorbed via the skin of the glans instead of the urethra. This can sometimes cause pains in the cavernous body and sometimes has a tendency to have no other effects whatsoever.

Vacuum pumps, which sound more like accessories in a sex store, also sometimes have a positive effect—not, however, the models that are used to pump out the cellar after a downpour. These vacuum pumps consist of plexiglass cylinders into which the penis is parked. The pump itself is found at the other end of the transparent tube. It's controlled by a button activated by the user—that is, the man whose penis is at this moment parked in the tube. On activation, a vacuum builds up in the cylinder, allowing the venous blood into the cavernous body and, as if by magic, resulting in an erection. Not a rock hard erection, but still rigid enough to guarantee a smile on the faces of both parties at breakfast the next day.

For the erection to stay once the vacuum pump has been removed, before the vacuum is turned off a penis ring—already awaiting its deployment inside the plexiglass cylinder—is slipped over the cavernous body. While we're here, let me just say that penis rings are an amazing invention! You can buy them in sex stores, online, or—pretty poor quality but at unbeatable prices—in the plumbing section of your local hardware store. They're inexpensive and can be a lot of fun when skillfully worked into lovemaking practices. But please, please remember one thing and spare a thought for the poor night-shift urologists at your local hospital: NO! STEEL!

How on earth could you think of such a thing? How foolish do you have to be to even try it? And why does it always have to be night shift when we are confronted with these questions?

Frank M. was in his mid-30s, wasn't scruffy or even bad looking—you could almost think you had a normal person standing in front of you... if it weren't for the fact that it was night in Emergency and, occasionally shaking our heads, we were viewing the sexual organ of a man who had had to make an emergency call to the fire department. What had happened?

Mr. M., in the course of indulging his little fetish, had acquired a new toy. As normal (pre)nuptial intercourse had become too routine, he had pepped up his love life with all kinds of accessories intended to heighten his sexual desires and those of his male and female partners. The new gem in his toy chest was a polished chrome ring as thick as a thumb. This ring was designed to slip over the penis and scrotum to restrict blood flow and thereby increase the intensity of the erection. When buying the ring, either Mr. M. wasn't focusing on the task at hand or, out of vanity, he chose a ring that was a size too large. After being installed, the gleaming adornment kept slipping off Mr. M.'s manhood until finally he was forced to seek a remedy. Instead of selecting a napkin ring from his granny's drawer or, with downcast eyes, facing anatomical realities and buying a smaller ring, Mr. M. came up with a brilliant idea. *If the mountain won't come to Muhammad then Muhammad must go to the mountain*, he probably thought as he injected a full load of saline solution into his scrotum.

Now it was so thick and swollen that the ring didn't move a fraction of an inch from its intended position. It was still in position after his mattress gymnastics were over and it was no longer needed. The next morning you could still plow a Siberian field in November with his erection, but now his penis was plum-colored and had doubled in size, which prompted Mr. M. to pay a visit to his local hospital.

In loose-fitting jogging pants, and slightly embarrassed by his unfortunate lot, he arrived at the urological unit. After obligatory attempts with soapy water proved to be woefully unsuccessful, all participants became quickly aware that given the material's strength, it would have to be countered with more appropriate techniques. By the time the fire department finally arrived, the poor patient, in ever-increasing pain, was equally embarrassed by and okay with the fact that this was a whole troop of four seasoned hulks who understandably, despite or maybe because of their entrance complete with fire department helmets and heavy-duty boots, were unable to hide a slight twitching around the corners of their mouths. Whether Mr. M. would have preferred to see a fireman's axe remains unknown. At any rate, he probably had a happier face when they walked in than the moment the hydraulic pliers appeared— the tool used for cutting through car wrecks to free road accident victims.

We quickly agreed to carry out the operation under anesthetic, more as an attempt to safeguard the patient's psyche than as a medical necessity. Besides, in whispered voices and with hands over our mouths, we nonpatients shared our doubts whether four firemen and a urologist were enough to guarantee the complete immobility that a patient needs in a situation like this!

As the patient dozed in Morpheus's arms, there was a flurry of activity in his southern zone. The men of the fire department were delighted with their green surgical gowns, which until recently they had only known from TV, and after donning them and putting the face masks over their helmets, they began to invent academic titles for each other. The patient, under the influence of the anesthetic, was fortunately not able to follow the heated discussion in the operating theater about the structural differences between and diverse material properties of car roofs and penis rings, or to hear that nobody really knew what would happen if a device with a clamping pressure of 10,000 kilos per square millimeter were to slip. As none of us seemed to want to precisely imagine the consequences, the officer in charge took heart and tool and chewed through the steel ring as if it were a damp breadstick. After a short round of applause, congratulations to the operator, and a few brief parting words, the troop returned to their station, enriched by a superb story.

IMPLANTS FOR MEN

The last resort of erection therapy is artificial: a cavernous body implant. When all else fails—when no pill in the world helps to bring even a minuscule amount of life to the penis, when injections and urethra probes don't cause even a twitch, when the vacuum pump just drones and the penis ring jams—then we have to get surgical!

Do you remember Stretch Armstrong, with its rubber arms and legs? To simplify, this type of artificial cavernous body implant consists of a filament—a wirelike fiber—enclosed in a silicone coating. These semi-rigid implants are roughly the size of a little finger and, depending on the afflicted member, about 6 to 8½ inches long (16 to 22 centimeters). This length includes not only what we consider to be the penis but also the invisible parts of the cavernous body that disappear into the depths behind the male pubic bone and are provided with a form of anchorage that helps during coitus. After all, a flagstaff isn't just poked into the topsoil but is properly, deeply fixed. Once the semi-rigid implants are surgically embedded along the penile tissues, you simply have to bend your dick upward on getting intimate with your partner. The advantage of these implants is that they're indestructible and the working principles are ingeniously simple: just plug and play.

PUMP AND PLAY

Somewhat more complicated are the pump implants. These consist of three components—reservoir, pump, and cavernous body—which have to be integrated. The reservoir is a plastic balloon about the size of an orange, which can be positioned near the bladder. It's connected by a system of tubes in the groin region to a pump in the scrotum. On waking up after the implant surgery, the patient will discover he has a third ball. The pump is activated by a press of the finger that allows liquid to flow from the balloon reservoir into the artificial cavernous body that the urologist has, hopefully, skillfully embedded in the distressed penis. And hey, presto! An erection occurs, not through romance but through hydraulics. Crazy world!

The beauty of multi-component implants is that the erection seems real. When the artificial cavernous body is filled, pressure in the penis increases and the patient feels proper sexual stimulation. The most recent models not only increase pressure in the cavernous body but also increase the length of the implanted tubes, which then not only erects the implant carrier's penis but also increases the length of his penis. Welcome to the third millennium.

The significantly more elaborate system makes these implants more susceptible to malfunctions than the plug and play method. Also, having three components means that more material is used and the risk of infection increases. However, many scientific studies have analyzed the quality of life of both patient and partner. All have shown that sex life and associated quality of life improve considerably—for *both* parties.

Finally, I'd like to return to the earlier definition of erectile dysfunction: that a diagnosis can be made only if the problem has existed for more than two months. Gentlemen, ladies, we're not erection machines, and if it still doesn't work out, it's not the end of the world.

seven

PREMATURE EJACULATION, AND WHAT YOU CAN DO ABOUT IT

THE DEFINITION OF premature ejaculation is no less
fraught than that of erectile dysfunction. International
experts have long discussed whether 60 seconds or
120 seconds is the measure of sexual fulfillment. In the
end the wisdom of Solomon prevailed, and the consensus
is: one to two minutes. Anyway, it's not only the length of
time that matters but, to a greater degree, the lack of control over ejaculation. Equally important is whether either
partner feels that the quality of their sexual life has been
impaired in any way. If all three issues coincide, *then* the
conditions are met for the diagnosis of premature ejaculation (PE). But let's be honest: if the intravaginal ejaculation
latency time (IELT) is three minutes or the patient can *just*
control the ejaculation—meaning that during sex he has
to wander out onto the balcony to water the flowers—then
even without a clear diagnosis, there's a problem that the
patient being treated needs to know about.

Every now and then I have patients in my practice about
their premature ejaculation because they can no longer

keep going for forty-five minutes but only twenty-five. These gentlemen also suffer from psychological strain—otherwise, they wouldn't have made an appointment. We presume that some 20 percent of men grapple with PE; the number of unrecorded cases is unknown.

Inherited or Acquired?

THE CAUSES OF premature ejaculation are often difficult to define. Very occasionally, hormonal disorders in testosterone metabolism or in the thyroid region can be diagnosed and treated. Considerably more often, nothing conspicuous can be found, so we assume an inherited or acquired disorder—which can be clarified in a few minutes by listening to the patient's story.

Here it's important to know if there is a difference in the problem between sexual intercourse and masturbation. When masturbating, if the distance to the finishing line is short, then the diagnosis of an inherited disorder is more likely. We speak of an *acquired disorder* when everything about the sex act was initially fine—excluding the wild sexual flings of youth—but problems gradually began to creep in. These acquired disorders in younger patients (up to about 40) are usually psychosomatic, meaning that something is wrong with their sex lives. After the age of 40, the prostate, the key male organ, pipes up to cause havoc. As most of the volume of ejaculate comes from the prostate and seminal vesicles, it's clear that acquired disorders after this age have little to do with the psyche and are more likely to be triggered organically.

Therapy

UP UNTIL RECENTLY there were few standard therapy options that patients could use to improve the situation. Since the 1960s, tips and tricks from the American research team Masters and Johnson have circulated, but their methods could be considered torture. There's the squeeze technique, whereby the woman, at the slightest signs of the ejaculatory greeting, pinches the glans with her fingernails so that the man, in the throes of agony, forgets to ejaculate. This extreme intervention has probably caused the demise of a number of marriages. The stop-start technique, in which the penis is withdrawn after two or three thrusts then a short break taken before resuming, is usually just as unhelpful: the ejaculation is now uncontrollable and quickly ends up in all its glory on the sheets. Either that or sex with a rhythm of one to two thrusts—stop, one to two thrusts, stop . . . — becomes so boring and tedious that knitting, TV, or the PlayStation will soon find more favor.

Topical therapy methods are more likely to be successful. *Topical* here means that the therapy takes place at a target location, in this case the man, or rather, his glans. Treatment comes in the form of a special condom with a reservoir filled with a gel-like substance that contains a low dose of local anesthetic such as lidocaine. When the condom is slipped on, the gel, warmed by body heat, becomes a thin liquid film that can be stroked over the glans. This reduces the sensitivity of the glans, meaning that things take a little longer than usual. Of course, after allowing a short time for the anesthetic to take effect, the condom can be removed. Great care should be taken to wipe off the residual film after it has taken effect, or the anesthetic will spread to the vaginal mucous membrane or clitoris region, having the same effects there—which are more than likely to prove rather counterproductive.

Besides condoms, you can also be prescribed ready-made ointments in a tube, but be careful with the dosage: the ointments are so effective that you could easily have a ring pierced right through your glans without shedding a single tear. There are also glans-numbing sprays that can be found on the internet or in specialist stores. These, however, don't always contain proper local anesthetics as active ingredients but rather substances that appear to work as a local anesthetic only later to be found lacking or ineffective.

A further option for premature ejaculation is a visit to a sexual therapist. Even though inherited disorders are certainly difficult to treat, an appointment could be worthwhile. Two prerequisites for successful sexual therapy, however, have to be fulfilled: you need a lot of patience and a large wallet.

ALPHA BLOCKERS: THE EJACULATORY REVERSE GEAR

If you put aside the differences between "inherited" and "acquired" and look instead, with an andrologist's inner eye, at "central" and "peripheral," then other possibilities emerge. As mentioned previously, the peripheral prostate and seminal vesicles belong to the ejaculatory system. The prostate is notorious for its bad behavior, and it spoils a not inconsiderable proportion of men's lives with annoying symptoms.

At the beginning of a man's life it's not even needed, and just loiters around in the pelvic zone. It has a purpose only if you want offspring. The prostate produces, among other things, food for sperm cells, and it ensures that the gooey, gel-like substrate that shoots out on ejaculation becomes fluid after a few minutes. Sperm in the uterus then have enough time to swim to the egg cell coming from the other direction. No sooner is the phase of wanting children over at around 40 than the prostate begins to grow and tighten, which can be extremely annoying both when having sex and when passing water.

One treatment that I prescribe for PE is related to this devil of an organ. With an alpha blocker—a medicinal inhibition of alpha receptors in the prostate and the neck of the bladder—the prostate's muscle cells become relaxed, reducing pressure in the gland. This has long been a known treatment for elderly patients with waterworks problems. These drugs can also be prescribed to other patients as off-label therapy to make use of their side effects.

Many patients receiving alpha blockers complain of ejaculation problems. Either their ejaculation is considerably weaker or it just comes as hot air. The ejaculate then often ends up in the bladder or doesn't even leave the prostate and the seminal vesicles. This happens because of the relaxation in the muscular portion of the prostate (and, in part, the bladder outlet), which causes a change in the pressure ratios in the urethra and prostate, which, in turn, results in a kind of ejaculatory reverse gear or, as the case may be, an idle state. If this happens, patients with peeing problems are not amused and the medication has to be exchanged. Luckily, there are a number of other candidates in this group of drugs, and you just have to try to find the right one. However, for patients suffering from organically based and/or peripheral premature ejaculation who have a problem with high pressure in the seminal ducts, this group of drugs can work miracles.

I remember well a patient who suffered from the maximum sentence: *ejaculatio ante portas*. This unfortunate guy couldn't enter his partner even for a few seconds but instead shot his load at the doorstep, as it were. Two days after his appointment, I received a joyful phone call about a full fifteen minutes of magical intercourse after taking the new medication. Incidentally, "off-label therapy" means that the safety of the medication for the purposes that we had prescribed it—for its side effects—hadn't been supported by research. Naturally, safety had been tested for its proper use, difficulties in passing water, or the medication couldn't have been prescribed at all. Off-label therapy also means that in some places even insured patients have to pay the costs.

MUSCLE TRAINING

The pelvic floor, the sacred cow of muscle groups! This muscle plate marks the lower borders of the abdominal region, is some 2 inches wide (5 centimeters), and consists of twenty-four different muscles, including two sphincter muscles: one for the gut and one for the bladder. You can figure out that the arrangement of its functions is complicated simply from the knowledge that we wake up in dry, clean sheets and don't need a college degree to go to the toilet without making a mess. In my student days, the lecturers were so fascinated by the subject of the pelvic floor that they almost went into raptures. I've since come to understand their enthusiasm.

As the pelvic floor is closely linked to the prostate and the seminal vesicles and is also deeply involved in ejaculation, it could also be one of the pitfalls of premature ejaculation. Viewing the pelvic floor as a mirror of the psyche is taking things a bit too far, but I'm fairly certain that the pelvic floor reacts to stress. Whether the constant need to urinate when about to take an exam or urge incontinence (overactive bladder) in women, the symptoms can often be improved by targeted relaxation of the pelvic floor area. One technique that can be helpful is progressive muscle relaxation, developed by Edmund Jacobson, which integrates the pelvic floor as a muscle group. You can find instructions on the internet or in well-stocked bookstores.

SHORT-LIVED HAPPINESS HORMONES

Alongside the peripheral causes are the central problems. When doctors say "central," they always mean the brain. A "central" problem probably just sounds better than a "brain problem" and takes some of the drama out of the equation. In the brain are a number of "centers"—areas where something happens. There is the respiratory center, which ensures that we don't stop breathing when we're asleep; there is an intestinal center that makes sure that breakfast is transported in the right direction and finds its way to the sewage system. And there is an ejaculation center, which makes sure that at the instant of utmost bliss, sperm sets off on its great journey.

The central regulation of ejaculation is dependent on the neurotransmitter serotonin—the happiness hormone. If there is too little serotonin locally, ejaculatory control is gone and the orgasm surges on like an unleashed hunting dog chasing a hare. In earlier days, antidepressants were prescribed as off-label therapy. In depression there can be significantly lower levels of serotonin at the point of effect (the brain). Nowadays there are countless selective serotonin reuptake inhibitors—SSRIs—for the pharmaceutical treatment of depression, which ensure that serotonin stays longer where it belongs, or rather, where its effects develop, namely, in the synaptic gap between two nerve cells. Lo and behold, a side effect of antidepressants often turned out to be delayed or even no ejaculation during sex. The off-label idea sprang to mind and patients with PE were prescribed antidepressants. Compared to the alpha blockers, the problem here is that centrally acting medications have to be taken continuously and for a long time to take effect. Sometimes the brain can get up to all sorts of mischief—especially the brains of the psychologically sound—and accordingly allow undesired side effects to emerge.

But here too the pharmaceutical industry has come up with something: SSRIs that influence serotonin *metabolism* are active only for a short time and don't have antidepressant effects. One such medication, dapoxetine, recently arrived on the market and is, as I write, the only medication approved in Germany for treating PE. It works well with some patients, not so well with others; sometimes it has side effects, sometimes none at all. It is definitely a treatment option if none of the abovementioned therapies work and a man's relationship begins to be put to the test. Once we know the patient tolerates the drug, we can start with higher dosages in order to give him a feeling of inner security. Once things get rolling and the man gets used to sex lasting a few minutes instead of seconds, the dosage can be gradually reduced in an attempt to become independent of the drug in the near future.

A DETOUR TO STEADY HAPPINESS

Premature ejaculation also has an orthomolecular therapy approach. The above-mentioned happiness hormone and neurotransmitter, serotonin, cannot be taken in drug form. The building blocks that the body needs to produce serotonin, however, can be. Serotonin is derived from tryptophan, one of the twenty amino acids that we consume daily. Today you can get it in capsules for the treatment of PE, but the supplement contains tryptophan in such small doses that I find it difficult to imagine that it can have an effect on ejaculation. Treatment with tryptophan, however, was used earlier for sleeping disorders and depressive mood swings in doses of up to 6,000 milligrams a day. If a patient with PE wishes to try out tryptophan, I usually recommend a gradual increase in dosage up to 3,000 to 4,000 milligrams per day in conjunction with magnesium citrate, which catalyzes the formation of serotonin via tryptophan.

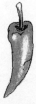

eight

TESTOSTERONE: THE STEAMROLLER OF HORMONES

TESTOSTERONE IS PRODUCED almost exclusively in the testicles. A tiny bit does come from the adrenal gland, which can be set aside for the time being. After puberty, this key male hormone ensures that a man is a man, at least as far as his surroundings and socialization allow. But at a certain age the testosterone-producing cells in the testicles start to dwindle and testosterone levels sink. Statistically, from the age of 40 on you have to make do with 1 percent less testosterone each year. This reduction in testosterone is a typical sign of aging and shouldn't be a drama—hair turns gray, testosterone levels sink. However, we tend to assume that older men's lower testosterone levels don't only have to do with reduced production in the testicles but are also linked to complications associated with other illnesses in old age. "Normal" for testosterone levels covers a pretty wide range. Normal for Mr. Miller can be eight times what it is for Mr. Smith. Both gentlemen probably lead normal lives, both own beautiful cars and maybe belong to a gym, without Mr. Miller having to think about sex all the time or having a huge erection when he sees a woman's bicycle, and without Mr. Smith constantly running into the corner for a good weep. Some people cope with low levels of testosterone, others with higher levels. Of course it makes sense for doctors to have "normal" reference levels for hormones as a guideline, but numbers are one thing—the symptoms of low testosterone levels are another.

Testosterone has physical, psychological, and sexual effects. Mostly you don't even notice that testosterone is there. You've become used to your level over the years. Problems only arise if your testosterone levels drop in a way that doesn't correspond to the aging process.

Often patients come to me with problems with their libido—a declining desire for sexual pleasure—and some also have erection disorders. And if there is such a thing as a typical testosterone patient, he is overweight and suffers from mood swings. There are many other testosterone-deficiency symptoms as well: a tendency to perspire, sleeping disorders, pains in the joints, fatigue, loss of strength, and skin changes, to name a few. The problem with the symptoms of testosterone deficiency is that they're so universal in nature that they don't necessarily mean you're suffering from a lack of testosterone. Everyone is tired sometimes, is in a bad mood, or sweats more than normal. Generally, however, the more points a patient scores on a testosterone questionnaire (ask your urologist for one), the more likely the cause is a hormonal problem. If that suspicion is supported by low, or even *too* low, testosterone levels in the blood, then the diagnosis is all the more likely.

For a complete diagnosis of low testosterone, further tests should be conducted to exclude a "central" source. The testosterone balance in the testicles is also governed by the brain—the hypothalamic-pituitary-adrenal axis... such a pleasing term. If the testicles are functioning well, the hormones from the brain—luteinizing hormone (LH) and follicle-stimulating hormone (FSH)—are relaxed and accordingly only register low levels in the bloodstream. (Both LH and FSH, by the way, originate in the pituitary gland.) If there are testosterone-related problems in the testicles, LH levels rise and stimulate the testicles to produce more testosterone. If testosterone levels and LH levels are low, the problem lies even higher up the hormonal hierarchy in the brain—in the hypothalamus. Here too hormonal disorders can begin that later result in reduced testosterone values. Last but not least, there is prolactin, which is also based in the pituitary gland. Prolactin is important for developing women's milk ducts during pregnancy and stimulates milk production after birth. The significance of prolactin in men is unknown, but its levels shoot up shortly after an orgasm and in times of stress.

A prolactinoma is probable with reduced testosterone levels and a simultaneous increase in prolactin. Prolactinoma is a prolactin-producing tumor that, when it grows, forces LH out of the pituitary, resulting in a testosterone deficiency. So far, so good? The beauty of prolactinomas is that they can sometimes be easily and effectively treated with just one pill a week and testosterone is back on track. Unfortunately, as they're easy to treat, prolactinomas are pretty rare.

When symptoms have been indicated as present by a questionnaire but normal or higher testosterone values have been recorded, further lab tests can provide a bit more clarity. The testosterone that is measured in the bloodstream is total testosterone—all the testosterone swimming around in the blood. Testosterone, however, can be found in free and bonded forms, although the active constituents can only be found in free testosterone. Sex hormone binding globulin (SHBG) is a protein that is mostly produced in the liver and that binds mainly to testosterone. The more SHBG and albumin that you have in your blood, the more testosterone will be bound and thus ineffective. This means that high concentrations of the bonding protein can produce the symptoms of deficiency together with normal to high testosterone readings. The proportions of free, effective testosterone can be detected by measuring SHBG and calculating from there.

Just to make things a little more complicated, there are also genetic tests that provide further information about testosterone. Measuring the CAG repeats (a sequence of three DNA bases—cytosine, adenine, and guanine—that appears multiple times) of Y chromosomes allows conclusions to be drawn about the potential exploitation of testosterone. Few CAG repeats means that the testosterone is less effective. In our practice, the CAG repeats tests, when necessary, are carried out by our geneticist. They seldom occur and are undertaken at the moment mostly in the interests of scientific research.

The Tiger in the Tank

AFTER THAT RATHER scientific introduction to the male hormone, let's return to andrological routine. If the symptoms of a testosterone deficiency are apparent and lab findings substantiate them, then we can initially try short-term testosterone therapy. Nowadays, there are a number of possible ways to raise testosterone levels in the blood. With my patients, I usually start with a gel that should be rubbed into the skin every day after the morning shower. If the symptoms arise from low testosterone levels, you can see an improvement very quickly. This becomes especially clear with a low score in questionnaires. In my opinion testosterone therapy together with questionnaires should be standard practice.

Even more impressive for me as a doctor—and for the patient—are the subjective changes we witness during treatment. More than once a grumbling, moaning whiner has morphed into a radiant, active, vivacious creature. The first changes can be expected within the first two weeks, which is how long we usually spend on testosterone treatment.

If the effects can be verified and the patient wants to continue treatment, then first more testing is done in order to plan mid-term and long-term therapy. This should definitely include tests to exclude the possibility of prostate cancer and breast cancer—yes, men can get breast cancer too. Prostate cancer is fundamentally testosterone-dependent. However, the old theory that administration of hormones triggers cancer has been completely discredited by numerous studies. I've even had prostate cancer patients who, after being cured, have been given testosterone under certain conditions and with regular control visits. This wouldn't have been possible ten years ago without my being on the receiving end of astonished looks from many of my colleagues.

Blood and liver values should also be within acceptable ranges, as testosterone is broken down in the liver. If the liver is playing up, testosterone often accumulates there, which can lead to an overdose. Maybe some of you have suffered the consequences of an overdose without realizing it—endurance athletes, for instance, particularly cyclists on the Tour de France, suddenly dropping from their saddles. Among other things, testosterone triggers an increase in the production of red blood corpuscles. This enables, in the medium and long term, an improvement in physical activity, as more oxygen is being supplied to the bloodstream. But if during long-term overdoses there are too many red cells in the blood and at the same time physical exertion causes a loss of liquid in the form of sweat, the blood's fluidity becomes increasingly compromised, and this can lead to circulation problems. This means that during testosterone therapy the composition of the blood should be regularly monitored.

If the patient suffers from sleep apnea, a disorder characterized by pauses in breathing during sleep, then a corrective has to be applied: testosterone therapy deepens sleep, and in theory the breathing pauses could intensify. Finally, concurrent medication should be reviewed, as some people don't always tolerate hormone therapy.

An important factor, especially with younger patients, is the influence of testosterone on their fertility. In the medium term, administration of hormones means that the testicles cease producing testosterone, which also results in a drop in sperm production. So testosterone can also make you infertile! Normally, the testicles resume sperm production after treatment has run its course, but it can take time and the resumption hasn't been completely supported by studies.

Low testosterone doesn't lead only to these direct deficiency symptoms. A number of studies in recent years have shown that too-low levels of testosterone can increase the risk of obesity, cardiovascular disorders, diabetes, and deterioration in fat metabolism, with all their accompanying problems. These diseases, clustered together as *metabolic syndrome*, are responsible today for more deaths than cancer. A few high-ranking scientists have stuck their necks out and claimed that people with low testosterone levels can prolong their lives by undergoing hormone therapy.

Still, treatment, especially of young patients, doesn't have to be and shouldn't be a permanent solution. Low levels of testosterone can be revived through physical activity and weight loss. Men's internal stomach fat—the stuff that gives you a beer belly—is hormonally pretty active and, by accumulating female sex hormones, inhibits testosterone. In this context in our practice I've often found that overweight and symptomatic testosterone-deficient patients become active during testosterone treatment, take up some sport or other, and lose weight. Once the stomach fat has been reduced to a state where testosterone levels no longer have an effect, the dosage can be slowly reduced so that the testicles can begin to crank up their own production processes. If necessary, this can be assisted, as off-label therapy, by antiestrogens. This will increase the concentrations of LH and FSH in the blood and support the body's own production of testosterone.

When It's Not a Testosterone Deficiency

WHAT HAPPENS WHEN the symptoms of a testosterone deficiency are there but blood tests don't support it and testosterone therapy doesn't seem to improve the situation? Either the symptoms have nothing to do with testosterone metabolism or the patient is simply tired or, for some reason or another, he doesn't feel like having sex. It's not that unusual.

The advantages and disadvantages of testosterone therapy, with all the hormonal transformations involved, have been discussed in the media for years. Patients, after acquiring some info on their own, come to our practice specifically to have their hormonal metabolism checked. Often the conviction that they have a hormone problem is so great that maybe the problem of not feeling like sex with their partner is pushed into the background.

On the other hand, their symptoms could have been caused not by a testosterone deficiency but rather by a lack of thyroid hormones. Thyroid deficiencies are pretty rare for men but by no means negligible. In our practice, we always recommend checking thyroid function during the initial round of tests.

From Testosterone Deficiency to Burnout Syndrome

ANOTHER CAUSE OF the described symptoms can be prolonged stress. Some researchers are convinced that the occupational burnout prominent nowadays also has its start in hormones. In this scenario, however, testosterone should be seen as a hanger-on and not the actual trigger. Stress can reduce testosterone levels, and low testosterone levels, in turn, lower resistance to stress. If someone is suffering from chronic stress, then the levels of the hormone cortisol—the stress hormone—increase. Cortisol is catabolic, which means that it breaks down proteins in the body (whereas testosterone is anabolic: it produces proteins, for example in the muscles of doped athletes). If during prolonged stress there is also a prolonged catabolic metabolic status, then everything that isn't nailed down will be metabolized. This includes proteinogenic components of blood that are not necessarily essential to life, such as the feel-good hormone serotonin, as well as noradrenaline and dopamine.

Noradrenaline is adrenaline's little sister. Besides having cardiovascular effects, it also has hormonal effects as a neurotransmitter enhancing alertness and focusing attention. Dopamine is the Swiss Army knife of neurotransmitters and is involved in mood, learning capacities, sleep, and motor functions, to name just a few things.

If cortisol has used up all these messenger substances— and we're talking just a few milligrams swimming around in the bloodstream—a huge, gaping, dark abyss opens up into which the patient falls with all the associated ailments. That's what burnout looks like at least from the perspective of a neurotransmitter. The problem is that the body, with the amino acids it gets from a steak, bread rolls, and maybe a salad, can't restore the feel-good hormones by itself.

Here, orthomolecular therapy can lend a hand. High doses of the amino acids tryptophan, phenylalanine, and tyrosine give the body the opportunity to assemble the substances that it has used up. Of course, in the early stages of burnout or other forms of extreme fatigue, it doesn't make sense just to gulp down large quantities of pills and powders. The fundamental problems—stress and the life situation—also have to be tackled, if need be with professional psychological assistance.

The point is that the intake of amino acids and nutrient supplements doesn't cancel much out, and that maybe a bit of self-determination can turn the situation around. For someone who doesn't feel good, fit, or happy, diagnosis and treatment are useful in possibly avoiding even more severe crises, whatever the problem ultimately is. Once testosterone values return to the lower normal range and treatment has improved the symptoms, we move into the off-label realm—lifestyle therapy, the costs of which are not covered by health insurers.

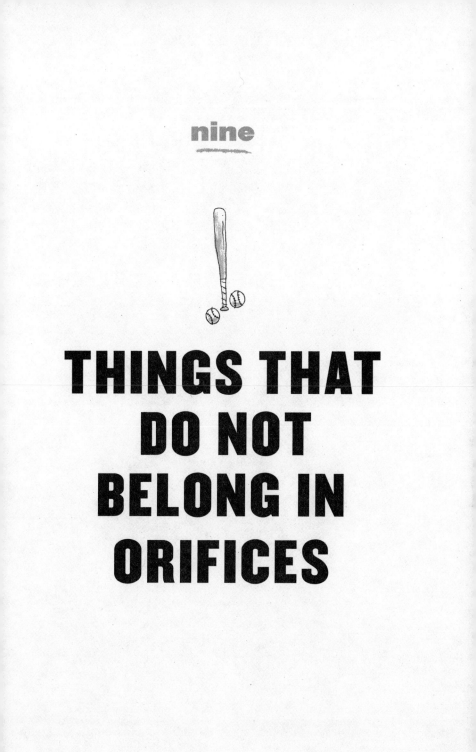

nine

THINGS THAT DO NOT BELONG IN ORIFICES

'M ON DUTY. It's Sunday morning. My rounds are over, and all the patients are more or less satisfied—I am, in any case. I'm strolling along the corridor of the hospital, almost bored, when my beeper drags me back to reality.

"The man doesn't want to tell me what's wrong with him, but judging by the way he's wiggling about, there's definitely something wrong with him," says the triage nurse from Emergency rather cryptically. My urological heart picks up a beat. It's the weekend; a man is prancing about in Emerg and doesn't dare say a word—it's definitely not kidney stones.

Curious as a kid at Christmas, I head to Emerg. I notice him immediately: mid-40s, small build, hasn't been to a barber for a while, and incredibly restless. Like an Energizer Bunny he's jiggling around the waiting room; it's almost making me dizzy just watching him. "Sit down now and tell me calmly what has happened," I order with all the doctor-like authority I can muster on a Sunday morning.

I've hardly managed to park him on a seat for a few seconds before he jumps up and continues his endless travels around the small room. "Okay, it was like this," he says, and launches into a chaotic monologue during which I manage to pick up a few words: "pot," "girlfriend gone," "a few too many beers," "I will never, ever do that again."

"Stop! You are sitting—or rather, *should* be sitting—in a hospital in Emergency. People don't usually come here just for fun. So, short answers please: What's wrong?"

"I shoved a dildo up my bum and now it's gone."

Okay, that's to the point. Respect. Somehow I'm still not quite sure of the reasons for his restlessness. "And you're trying to shake the thing out, right?" I ask, my head orbiting from watching him circling the room.

"No," he replies. "I put in new batteries yesterday and the thing is still running." *Now it's getting interesting*, I think, and begin to develop a bit of sympathy for the unfortunate sex fiend.

"And the thing won't come out the natural way?"

"Just the opposite, dammit. The thing is slowly working its way up my guts. This morning it was tingling beneath my pelvis, and now it's clearly arrived to the left of my stomach."

If we wait a little longer and the batteries hold out, maybe we can contact the ear, nose, and throat specialist, I think, but then the seriousness of the situation gets a grip on me. If the torpedo-shaped love buzzer continues its trip through the gentleman's intestines, it could end up doing serious damage to his guts and then the brown stuff will *really* hit the fan. So, time to roll up sleeves and get the thing out. But how?

For the first attempt, the poor soul is placed on a uro-logical examination chair. While my assistant tenderly massages the abdomen from above, trying to encourage the offending object to seek the light of day, I try from the other end, using specula and long pliers, to grasp the wretched thing and guide it out. After passing a 15-inch-long (40-centimeter) tool through the sphincter muscle, I cannot deny a certain feeling of claustrophobia. "Okay, this is getting us nowhere. Let's try *per vias naturales*," I suggest.

Without batting an eye, the man gulps down 3 liters—almost a gallon—of that irrigating solution that patients usually take before bowel surgery, leaving the gut as clean as a whistle. As soon as the liquid takes effect, the object *should* sweep through the rectum like a white-water raft with three silver batteries as screaming passengers, and the dildo should land with a resounding clunk in the pan amid a streaming torrent. The outcome after two long hours: plenty of software, no hardware. We're as disappointed as when we lost our soccer match against the team from cardiology, but we rattle our brains about how we can put an end to this slithery customer's game. Okay, sharpen up the knives!

While I'm explaining the surgical procedure, the thought creeps into my mind that we'll be working with electronic scalpels that cut and seal small blood vessels at the same time. My university physics course was a long time ago and I don't want the gentleman to sign the consent form if there's a chance that when electricity meets electricity, there might be an almighty short circuit in his bowels, resulting in the cleaning staff having to painstakingly scrape the last few feet of his digestive tract from the walls. So we might as well wait until the batteries have given up the ghost.

The doughty patient has been in our care for six hours and is now visibly distraught. "What am I supposed to tell my family? I mean, about having to have an operation," he whines. I tell him that I can easily explain that part of the story to his loved ones—not, however, how the dildo got there.

At some stage even the liveliest Energizer Bunny wears out. This the man imparts with a raised hand and a tired "I think it's stopped." The anesthetist puts the patient to sleep after giving him a sizable dose of relaxant so that all muscles, be they responsible for arms or for clean underwear, are immobilized. One final attempt at wrestling the stubborn object from the greedy clutches of the rectum and lo and behold, thanks to the anesthetically and pharmaceutically induced relaxation, the sphincter muscles are so loose that you could almost fish the pink metallic, blinking torpedo out of the depths of the rectum with your bare hands. "Oh, it's a boy!" declares the anesthetist.

SINCE BECOMING A urologist, I have time and again been reminded that there are no boundaries to the scope of lovemaking. I consider it a privilege that my patients have so much trust in me and often allow me insights deep into their intimate lives, sometimes a bit *too* deep for my liking. However, the more I know, the more I can picture a patient's situation and develop treatment strategies that can help as quickly and efficiently as possible. As long as their sexual practices don't harm anyone, then, of course, it's none of my business what the Millers or Smiths or any other couple do in their bedrooms, alone or together. Nevertheless, sometimes I do wonder.

There was, for instance, the gentleman who confessed that he could only do it when he was "electrified." I took this to be metaphorical until the physical examination revealed third-degree burns to his scrotum. "Electrified" for this guy meant at least 12 volts. Up till then he'd managed to make do with the small block batteries from a model car remote control; now to get things going he had to plug into a proper car battery.

Often the urethra is the object of sexual stimulation. On the one hand, this is not totally incomprehensible because the urethra, as a tissue well supplied by nerves, belongs to a man's sexual tackle. On ejaculation, sperm shoots through the urethra, creating pressure waves that are felt all along its length, making this a considerable part of the orgasmic experience. On the other hand, the urethral mucous membrane is a devil of an organ. Even if it's only slightly injured, the result can be prolonged disruptions, irritation, and scarring. A badly placed bladder catheter can lead to repercussions lasting many years. I remember a number of hospital patients who had to have surgery because of urethral stenosis, a narrowing or blockage of the urethra, which is why I can't help pulling a face whenever I hear about what men do to themselves and their urethras. For instance, cock stuffing, in which men over the years feed thin surgical metal rods down their urethra until it expands so much that another man can stuff his aroused penis in the other man's urethra.

In Berlin I had a patient in Emergency who got satisfaction from matches. So far, so good. Stick the match in the urethra, light it, and wait as long as you can before snuffing the match... but I wouldn't recommend it.

Two particular stories on the subject of urethral arousal have especially stuck with me from my time at the Charité in Berlin...

SOMEONE WHO BUYS a car and later discovers he can't afford it is being rash. Someone who invites a woman on holiday even though he only met her that day is being very rash. Someone who feeds something into his urethra without thinking about how to retrieve it is being *extremely* rash. And this first story is of a man who, wandering through the woods shortly before Christmas, stuck an evergreen bough into his urethra with the intention of masturbatory pleasure.

We'd already heard stories of doped bodybuilders who, thanks to veterinary doses of testosterone and out of pure horniness, are supposed to have tried to penetrate the outlets of vending machines. How someone makes the jump to Christmas decorations, however, remains a mystery. According to the gentleman, the insertion itself was no problem, but on trying to extract it, the pine bough became snagged.

So there the man was, standing bowlegged in the hospital, bits of greenery dangling from his pants and blood dripping onto his shoes. With legs wide apart, he took tiny steps, reminding one of the grace of a Japanese geisha crossed with the brawn of an Albanian construction worker. Every millimeter the bough moved, to the left or right, up or down, caused excruciating agony. Already, shortly after his arrival, the hospital grapevine was in full swing and details of his case had been passed to all emergency stations with the most florid descriptions. Now there was whispering of whether we should bring along some candles, or at least some baubles or candy canes, to make the situation a bit more relaxed and Christmassy. That would have been his death sentence.

After a generous dose of an opiate painkiller, that was the end of all things Christmassy. Much more pressing was the answer to the question of how to get a stick out of the penis without turning the urethra into flesh-colored tinsel. It's often said that a urethra never forgets. A badly placed catheter, a soccer ball in the scrotum, or slipping onto the crossbar of a bike can be enough for a season ticket to the local urologist for urethral slitting. A cautious approach was called for if the gentleman ever wanted to stand next to his peers at the urinal again. A colleague had, in the meantime, joined me, and together we considered the available options. Of course under anesthetic, we could have given the stick a hefty tug, but the man's urethra would then be history. On top of that, had we reverted to barbaric forms of treatment, as we term them, pine needles might have lodged in the penile tissue and caused a whole heap of problems. Maybe the previous day a fawn had peed on this particular bough before it was rudely plucked from the tree as a masturbation aid, and then the sorry pine fetishist would have fawn's pee plus some sort of weird fawn germs in his cavernous body. As a urologist I don't even want to consider the consequences...

After asking the patient about the probable length of his wooden ornament (25 centimeters—that's 10 inches!), we opted for the push-pull method. The man, together with his portion of the pine tree, was taken to the operating theater and, after a few compassionate words, given an anesthetic. While slumbering in a parallel universe he was placed in the lithotomy position: lying down, legs up and apart, with the aid of a gynecological chair. My colleague sought out and found the other opening in the man's south, into which, incidentally, you can also inadvisedly introduce objects like pine boughs. From here he could feel the prostate, which didn't appear to have been pierced by pine needles. From the upper opening I cautiously pushed the small branch deeper and deeper into the forbidden zone until my colleague bellowed loudly: "Stop!"

By now the branch had been almost completely swallowed and we had to use a bladder examination device. With a pair of small forceps, I could get a good grip on the stick and continue to push it until the other end had reached the bladder. After a routine sectio alta—an incision in the lower abdomen—we were soon greeted by a strange evergreen growth not common in this region. Now we could completely withdraw the offending object through the open bladder without laying a finger on the urethra. A quick look through the maltreated urethra with the cystoscope revealed that, fortunately, the tube had only mild signs of piercing. After surgery the man was taken to the ward, where, just to be on the safe side, all Christmas decorations were placed well out of sight.

WHAT WE HAVE had so far: a dildo up the backside, a pine bough up the urethra, and a number of different penis rings. On top of these, and the order is random, my colleagues and I have recovered the following everyday objects: a pencil (as an erection aid), a paint brush (badger's hair, da Vinci model), a pearl necklace (belonging to Grandma), a telephone cable (coiled), plaster (initially liquid, then not), and maggots (alive); paper clips, pen refills, and felt-tip-pen caps (the urethra office); wall hooks, nails, and snap hooks (the urethra workshop); and a plastic action figure (crawling). It seems almost impossible to top this list, but Mr. K. managed to do so.

"No, you don't stuff that into your urethra" is a sentence that you could assume doesn't need to be said, like "Please don't play in the yellow snow," "Don't drink the paint stripper," or "Please wear your seat belt in the car." Mr. K. obviously wasn't listening. This is what happened.

A man, mid-30s, came to the practice complaining of a slight burning sensation when passing water. For a urologist, this is a common symptom to hear about. The cause this time, however, was rather unusual. After the routine inquiry into the medical history hadn't revealed anything conspicuous, the ultrasound came up with the answer.

The sonogram of a full bladder is pitch black. An empty bladder is difficult to discern, at most a baffling form the size of an orange in various shades of gray. Mr. K.'s bladder— or rather, where the bladder should have been—appeared on the monitor as a large glossy white shape, as if someone had scanned a snowball the size of a grapefruit. So, where did we go from here?

I suggested taking X-rays and the patient consented. On the plates was the image of a fist-sized, 100 percent radiopaque raspberry projecting from the lesser pelvis. "Aha! We have found something that doesn't belong," I began, "and this something is pretty large. Do you have any suggestions as to how it got there?"

"Ah, yes... They must be the steel balls from the workshop, the ones I pushed up my urethra last month."

I remained silent and glanced, perplexed, out the window. In disbelief, I looked back at Mr. K. and then again out of the window. Then again at the X-ray, the window, and Mr. K. Somehow the comment, the X-ray plate, and the story that was just beginning to emerge in my mind didn't match the concept of human beings that I had developed over the years and that up to a few moments earlier I'd still had. "Okay..." I gathered myself. "Slowly and from the beginning. Which workshop? No, a different question. Why have you got hundreds of balls the size of .45 Magnum bullets... Er, no, how did you..."

I was a little lost about what to write in the outpatient file. Then I said something that always works: "Just explain what happened." And Mr. K. cheerfully launched into his story.

"Okay. I found a big sack full of steel balls from an abandoned warehouse in the workshop—they'd been set aside for disposal. I took them home and stored them there. Last month I was relaxing in the tub, and I asked myself, *What would happen if I stuck one of them into my penis?* Then suddenly there it was inside and it didn't hurt a bit."

"Yes, obviously. And then?" I asked incredulously.

"Then I was surprised that the ball didn't come out, and I put another one in. Then another, and another. Eventually, there was a *plop* in my stomach and it tickled a bit."

"Yes, congratulations! You were witnessing the balls passing through your prostate and popping up into your bladder," I said, trying to give him an understanding of the anatomical realities of the male urinary tract.

"Yes, exactly! And the tickling sensation was so pleasant that I fed in all the remaining balls."

"When I look at the small clusters of raspberries in your bladder, I'd say there are about three hundred balls that you must have painstakingly massaged along the urethra. Is that about right?"

"Four hundred twenty-seven," Mr. K. reported proudly.

I advised him to keep away from airport security until after the operation if he wanted to avoid stupid questions.

The evening when we surgically opened his bladder, we collected from his bladder bags full of industrially manufactured, highly polished steel balls with a diameter of some one-third of an inch (8 millimeters). Four hundred twenty-seven, to be precise.

INDEX

INDEX

turmeric, 112
TURP (transurethral resection of the
prostate), 79
tyrosine, 198

U
ultrasound: ovaries examination,
129; prostate cancer treatment,
93–94; prostate examination,
71, 73, 89
underwear, 105–6
urethra: anatomy, 36; genital
warts and, 49; infertility from
infections in, 54; male vs.
female lengths, 98; nonspecific
infections, 53; sexual arousal
from, 205–6
urine. See bladder capacity issues

V
vacuum pumps, 27, 169
varicoceles, 121
vasectomy: advantages, 143; costs
vs. the pill, 144–45; description,
142; lack of side effects, 68,
142–43; mixed antiglobulin
reaction (MAR), 146–49;
prevalence, 144; reversal
operation, 143–44, 145–46

veins, 42
Viagra, 62, 107, 163. *See also*
phosphodiesterase 5 (PDE5)
inhibitors
vitamin C, 110
vitamin D, 50, 110–11
vitamin E, 59

W
webbed penis, 26
women: cervical cancer, 49;
chlamydia, 54; contraceptive
pill, 139–40, 144–45; fallopian
tubes, 54, 130–31; ovaries, 129,
132. *See also* bladder infections;
fertility; infertility

Y
young men: acquired premature
ejaculation, 178; erectile
dysfunction, 155–56, 164–66;
familiarity with penis, 21–23;
penis length dissatisfaction, 32;
prostate cancer, 86; prostate
problems, 79–81; testosterone
therapy and fertility, 194–95